FRYE'S
2000
NURSING
BULLETS

NCLEX-RN

Third Edition

FRYE'S 2000 NURSING BULLETS

NCLEX-RN

Third Edition

Charles M. Frye, RN
Director
Professional Development Systems
Long Beach, California

Springhouse Corporation
Springhouse, Pennsylvania

Staff

EXECUTIVE DIRECTOR, EDITORIAL
Stanley Loeb

SENIOR PUBLISHER, TRADE AND TEXTBOOKS
Minnie B. Rose, RN, BSN, MEd

ART DIRECTOR
John Hubbard

CLINICAL CONSULTANT
Susan Galea, RN, MSN

EDITOR
Nancy Priff

COPY EDITOR
Barbara Hodgson

DESIGNERS
Stephanie Peters (Associate Art Director), Cindy Marczuk

COVER ILLUSTRATION
Cindy Marczuk

MANUFACTURING
Deborah Meiris (director), Anna Brindisi, Kate Davis, T.A. Landis

PRODUCTION COORDINATOR
Caroline Lemoine

Printed in the United States of America. For more information, write Springhouse Corporation, 1111 Bethlehem Pike, P.O. Box 908, Springhouse, PA 19477-0908.

NCLEXBTS - 040396

A member of the Reed Elsevier plc group

**Library of Congress
Cataloging-in-Publication Data**

Frye, Charles M.
Frye's 2000 nursing bullets NCLEX-RN/Charles M. Frye—3rd ed.
  p. cm.
    1. Nursing—Examinations, questions, etc. 2. Nursing—Outlines, syllabi, etc. I. Title. II. Title: Frye's two thousand nursing bullets for NCLEX-RN. III. Title: 2000 nursing bullets for NCLEX-RN. IV. Title: Two thousand bullets for NCLEX-RN.
    [DNLM: 1. Nursing—examination questions. WY 18 F948f 1994]
RT55.F79 1994
610.73'076—dc20
DNLM/DLC   93-44756
ISBN 0-87434-699-1   CIP

Preface

I remember in great detail preparing to take the state licensing examination for registered nurses. Of all the memories I associate with that event, the most vivid is my frantic search through the bookstores for the "right" review book that would provide answers to the test. I did not have the time and did not want to spend all my waking hours reading one of those 500-page review books. But nothing else was available—until now.

This book is different from the other review books you've seen or used. You're holding 2,000 nursing bullets—concise information that provides answers to questions not only on the upcoming NCLEX-RN, but also on the NCLEX-PN, Commission on Graduates of Foreign Nursing Schools (CGFNS) test, and any other nursing examination. How do these bullets work for you? They're concentrated nursing facts, stated in one or two sentences that are free of unnecessary or obscure words.

Test-question writers can create lengthy and time-consuming situations, provide minute (but not necessarily meaningful) details, and ask tricky questions that any of us can misunderstand. But they can't change nursing facts. These 2,000 nursing bullets are just that—facts. They are the answers you need for test questions.

Passing the examination is a necessary step in the licensing process, and you must be prepared for it. This book can help you meet that challenge.

Good luck.

Charles M. Frye, RN

How to use this book

Frye's 2000 Nursing Bullets NCLEX-RN, Third Edition, is designed to help you review for the NCLEX-RN effectively and efficiently. This book gives you nursing information that remains true in every clinical situation and setting, and these are the very facts that test-question writers must draw on in devising the test.

Use these suggestions to get the most from this unique book:

- Read the introduction to prepare for computerized adaptive testing, learn about the NCLEX-RN test plan, and develop effective test-taking strategies.

- Study the key facts as they are presented in random order. You'll realize two benefits from this approach: You'll master essential data in psychiatric, pediatric, maternal, and medical-surgical nursing (as well as the important concepts in nursing fundamentals), and you'll prepare yourself for the new computerized NCLEX-RN because it also presents questions at random.

- Review groups of nursing bullets throughout the day. Because this book is compact and easy to carry, you can take it with you wherever you go and review a few bullets whenever you have a spare minute—for example, when waiting for class to begin, during a break between labs, or while riding the bus or train.

- Use the book to create questions to quiz your study partner or members of your study group.

No matter how you choose to use this versatile book, you'll find that each nursing bullet is brief, easy to read, and free of clinical situations and excess wording. You'll find that you'll easily remember and identify the facts, no matter what form they take on the test. Because each bullet has been reviewed by a clinical expert, you can be sure that all the information is up-to-date and clinically accurate.

You've spent years studying to become a nurse and months preparing for the NCLEX-RN. Now, with *Frye's 2000 Nursing Bullets NCLEX-RN*, Third Edition, you can take this last step to licensure with confidence.

Introduction

In the United States, if you want to work as a registered nurse, you need a license from the nursing licensure authority in the state where you plan to practice. To get a license, you need to pass the National Council Licensure Examination for Registered Nurses (NCLEX-RN). This book will help you do just that. Its 2,000 bullets of nursing facts will expand and reinforce your nursing knowledge base. And this introduction will prepare you for the exam by describing the new computerized adaptive testing system, explaining the NCLEX-RN test plan, and providing effective test-taking strategies.

Scheduling your test

To schedule your NCLEX-RN, apply to your state board of nursing for testing. When your application is approved, the Educational Testing Service Data Center will send you an Authorization to Test and will advise you to make an exam appointment at one of 200 Sylvan Technology Centers throughout the country.

When scheduling your NCLEX-RN, remember that the test takes up to 5 hours and is offered 15 hours daily, Monday through Saturday, and sometimes on Sunday. The Sylvan Technology Center will schedule you for testing within 30 days of your call (or within 45 days for retesting). If you need to reschedule your exam appointment, call the Sylvan Technology Center at least 3 days beforehand.

Understanding computerized adaptive testing

Since April of 1994, the NCLEX-RN has been a computerized test. It requires you to answer sufficient questions of various difficulty levels to demonstrate minimum competence as an entry-level nurse. It is adaptive because it selects harder or easier questions based on your response to previous questions. For example, if you answer a medium-level question correctly, the computer will pose a more difficult question next. But if you answer incorrectly, it will choose an easier one.

The test bank includes thousands of questions categorized by difficulty level and the NCLEX-RN test plan. From this bank, the computer continues to pull questions until you demonstrate competence in all parts of the test plan. Therefore, each test is different and may require 75 to 265 questions to complete.

Before the test, a proctor will help you get started at a computer terminal. Then the test will begin with brief instructions and a practice session of 15 questions. During the practice session and the test, use only the space bar (to move the cursor to the four answer options) and the enter key (to select your answer). To avoid unintentional answers, the computer will ask you to confirm your answer selection by striking the enter key again.

During the test, the computer will display one question at a time. If a case study is included, it will appear to the left of the question. Consider each question carefully. Then press the space bar to move to the option that best answers the question. To record your answer, press the enter key twice. Because the computer does not let you skip questions or return to previous items, you must answer every question until the test ends.

The testing period includes a mandatory 10-minute break after 2 hours and an optional break 90 minutes after testing resumes.

Understanding the NCLEX-RN test plan
The NCLEX-RN test plan classifies questions by the five steps of the nursing process and the four categories of client needs. Each test question reflects one nursing process step and one client needs category.

Nursing process steps
The nursing process is a five-step method of performing nursing care. On the NCLEX-RN test, each nursing process step carries equal weight and accounts for 20% of the test questions.

- Assessment refers to forming a data base by gathering subjective and objective information about a patient.
- Analysis, or nursing diagnosis, refers to identifying actual or potential health problems based on assessment findings.
- Planning refers to establishing goals to meet the patient's needs and developing strategies for achieving those goals.

- Implementation refers to performing actions that accomplish the patient's established goals.
- Evaluation refers to measuring the extent of goal achievement.

Client needs categories

Client needs categories are based on data from a major nursing job survey. On the NCLEX-RN test, each category accounts for a varying percentage of the test questions.

- Physiologic integrity refers to meeting the physiologic needs of a patient with a life-threatening or recurring condition (or one at risk for complications or adverse effects of treatments) by providing care, reducing risks, and promoting physiologic adaptation and comfort. This category accounts for 42% to 48% of the test.
- Safe, effective care environment refers to promoting environmental safety, providing effective care, assuring quality, and performing treatments and procedures safely and effectively. This category accounts for 25% to 31% of the test.
- Health promotion and maintenance refers to meeting the patient's needs by promoting growth and development, self-care, support system integrity, and disease prevention and early treatment. This category accounts for 12% to 18% of the test.
- Psychosocial integrity refers to meeting the patient's psychosocial needs during times of stress or crisis by promoting coping skills and adaptation throughout the life cycle. This category accounts for 9% to 15% of the test.

Studying for the exam

To study for the NCLEX-RN as effectively as possible and enhance your ability to retain pertinent information, follow these study tips.

- Familiarize yourself with all exam topics.
- Answer as many practice questions as possible. (You and a study partner may want to use this book's bullets to develop questions for each other.)

- Understand the parts of a test question. On the NCLEX-RN, each multiple-choice question has a stem (the question itself) and four options: a key (correct answer) and three distractors (incorrect answers). A brief case study may precede any question.
- Use additional study guides as resources, such as *American Nursing Review for NCLEX-RN*, if desired.
- Organize a study group with other nursing students or take an NCLEX review course.
- Ask a colleague or nursing instructor to clarify unfamiliar or complex material.

Planning for the exam
Remember that the NCLEX-RN poses certain physical demands. To ensure your best test performance, use these pointers to help you plan for the exam—and cope with these demands.

- Schedule your test appointment at a testing center near your home, if possible. Before the test, assess the parking facilities and determine travel time.
- Make reservations well in advance at a hotel near the testing center if you must travel a long distance.
- Schedule your test appointment to take advantage of your peak-performance time.
- Avoid late-night, last-minute cramming. Obtain sufficient sleep the night before the test.
- Eat a well-balanced meal before the test.
- Wear layers of clothes that can be removed, as needed, to maintain warmth and comfort.
- Take your Authorization to Test and two forms of identification with signatures (including one photographic identification) to the testing center. You cannot take the exam without them.
- Use simple relaxation techniques, such as progressive relaxation, during the test to reduce anxiety.

Developing test-taking skills

Knowing the facts is *not* all you need to pass the NCLEX-RN. You also need to know how to take the test. To sharpen your test-taking skills, review these guidelines.

- Check case studies closely for information needed to answer the question correctly.

- Look for clue words, such as *best, first, most,* and *not* in the question's stem. These words, which may be highlighted, aid in selecting the correct answer.

- Imagine the correct response when reading the stem. If it appears as one of the four options, it is probably the correct one.

- Read every question—and all four of its options—carefully before making your final selection.

- Reread the stem and options when two options seem equally correct; look again for clues or differences that can help you select the correct answer. When in doubt, make an educated guess. Remember: You cannot skip questions.

- Do not panic if a question covers an unfamiliar topic. Draw on your knowledge of similar problems and nursing principles to help eliminate options and increase the chance of choosing the correct answer.

- Take your time and pace yourself. Do not spend excessive time on any one question.

- Do not be distracted by other candidates or the apparent length of their tests. Keep in mind that each test is individualized.

- Use break periods to rest your mind and body, for example, by eating a small snack, stretching, or doing relaxation exercises.

A note to foreign nurse graduates

If you were educated in a foreign country, you must meet the requirements of the state board of nursing in the state where you plan to practice. Most states require a certificate from the Commission on Graduates of Foreign Nursing Schools (CGFNS) before you take the NCLEX-RN.

Eligibility requirements for the CGFNS examination include successful completion of secondary education; a valid, current nursing license in the country in which you were educated; and graduation from a well-balanced, 2-year (or longer) nursing education program in a government-approved school.

The CGFNS examination tests your nursing knowledge and English proficiency. Its nursing portion follows the NCLEX-RN test plan and reliably predicts success on NCLEX-RN. Its English portion consists of written and listening sections. Its results reach you by mail 8 to 10 weeks after the test; passage of the test earns you a CGFNS certificate.

You can obtain application forms and the CGFNS Guidebook for Applicants through U.S. embassies in foreign countries, national nurses' associations, and the CGFNS at 3600 Market Street, Philadelphia, PA 19104-2651. The Guidebook for Applicants presents eligibility requirements, application procedures, fees, and suggestions for CGFNS test preparation.

• A child in Bryant's traction who is under age 3 or 30 lb (13.5 kg) should have the buttocks slightly elevated and clear of the bed. The knees should be slightly flexed, and the legs should be extended at a right angle to the body.

• Unlike false labor, true labor produces regular, rhythmic contractions, abdominal discomfort, no change in fetal movement, progressive fetal descent, bloody show, and progressive cervical effacement and dilation.

• Pernicious anemia results from failure to absorb vitamin B_{12} in the gastrointestinal (GI) tract and causes primarily GI and neurologic signs and symptoms.

• In a patient with hypokalemia (serum potassium level below 3.5 mEq/liter), presenting signs and symptoms include muscle weakness and arrhythmias.

• According to Kübler-Ross, the five successive stages of death and dying are denial, anger, bargaining, depression, and acceptance.

• Criteria for brain death vary from state to state but typically include unresponsiveness to painful stimuli, absence of spontaneous respiration or muscle movement, loss of brain stem function (as evidenced by fixed, dilated pupils and absence of reflexes), and a flat electroencephalogram (EEG).

• To help a mother break the suction of her breast-feeding infant, the nurse should teach her to insert a finger at the corner of the infant's mouth.

• A patient with a pressure sore should consume a high-protein, high-calorie diet, unless contraindicated.

• Creatine phosphokinase (CPK-MB) levels are used to assess tissue damage in myocardial infarction (MI).

• After a 12-hour fast, the normal fasting blood glucose level ranges from 70 to 100 mg/dl.

- A blood pressure cuff that is too narrow can cause a falsely elevated blood pressure reading.

- A blood pressure cuff that is too wide can cause a falsely decreased blood pressure reading.

- A patient with digitalis toxicity may report diplopia, blurred vision, light flashes, and yellow-green halos around images.

- The primary nurse is responsible for coordinating and evaluating the patient's care from admission to discharge.

- When preparing a single injection for a patient who takes regular and NPH insulin, the nurse should draw the regular insulin into the syringe first because it is clear and can be measured more accurately than the NPH insulin, which is turbid.

- *Anuria* refers to a daily urine output of less than 100 ml.

- In remittent fever, the body temperature varies over a 24-hour period but remains elevated.

- Rhonchi are the rumbling sounds heard on lung auscultation; they are more pronounced during expiration than during inspiration.

- *Gavage* refers to forced feeding, usually through a gastric tube (a tube passed into the stomach by way of the mouth).

- A taxonomy of nursing diagnoses has been formulated by the North American Nursing Diagnosis Association (NANDA). It classifies diagnoses by nine human response patterns: exchanging, communicating, relating, valuing, choosing, moving, perceiving, knowing, and feeling.

- To help venous blood return in a patient in shock, the nurse should elevate the patient's legs no more than 45 degrees. (This procedure is contraindicated in a patient with a head injury.)

- According to Maslow's hierarchy of needs, physiologic needs (air, water, food, shelter, sex, activity, and comfort) have the highest priority.

- Checking the identification band on a patient's wrist is the safest and surest way to verify a patient's identity.

- A patient's safety is the priority concern in developing a therapeutic environment.

- According to the Code for Nurses developed by the International Council of Nurses, the nurse must take appropriate action to safeguard the patient when the patient's care is endangered or jeopardized by the actions of a co-worker.

- The difference between the apical and radial pulse rates, when taken simultaneously by two nurses, is the pulse deficit.

- The nurse should schedule postural drainage before meals or 2 to 4 hours after meals to reduce the patient's risk of vomiting.

- Blood pressure can be measured directly by intra-arterial insertion of a cannula connected to a pressure-monitoring device.

- A positive Kernig's sign occurs when an attempt to flex the hip of a recumbent patient produces painful spasms of the hamstring muscle and resistance to further leg extension at the knee.

- In a patient with a fractured femur and displacement, treatment begins with reduction and immobilization of the affected leg.

- Herniated nucleus pulposus (intervertebral disk) most commonly occurs in the lumbar and lumbosacral regions.

- *Laminectomy* refers to the surgical removal of the herniated portion of an intervertebral disk.

• Surgical treatment of a gastric ulcer includes severing the vagus nerve (vagotomy) to reduce the amount of gastric acid secreted by the gastric cells.

• *Flight of ideas* refers to an alteration in thought processes characterized by skipping from one topic to another, unrelated topic.

• *La belle indifference* refers to the lack of concern for a profound disability, such as blindness or paralysis, that may occur in a patient with a conversion disorder.

• In an infant, a bulging fontanelle is the most significant sign of increasing intracranial pressure.

• With mild anxiety, a person's ability to perceive may increase.

• With moderate anxiety, a person's ability to perceive and concentrate decreases. The person is selectively inattentive (focuses on immediate concerns), and the perceptual field narrows.

• A patient with a phobic disorder uses self-protective avoidance as the ego defense mechanism.

• In a patient with anorexia nervosa, the highest treatment priority is correction of nutritional and electrolyte imbalances.

• Memory loss is the most common symptom of Alzheimer's disease.

• A patient's blood lithium level must be monitored regularly (usually once a month) because of the narrow margin between therapeutic and toxic levels. A level above 1.5 mEq/liter is considered toxic.

• *Valsalva's maneuver* refers to forced exhalation against a closed airway, as when taking a deep breath, blowing air out, or bearing down.

- Early signs and symptoms of alcohol withdrawal include anxiety, anorexia, tremors, and insomnia. They may begin up to 8 hours after the last alcohol intake.

- Al-Anon is a support group for families of alcoholics.

- The nurse should not administer chlorpromazine hydrochloride (Thorazine) to a patient who has ingested alcohol because it may cause oversedation and respiratory depression.

- Vital organ perfusion is seriously compromised when the mean arterial pressure falls below 60 mm Hg and the systolic blood pressure falls below 80 mm Hg.

- Lidocaine hydrochloride (Xylocaine) is the drug of choice for reducing premature ventricular contractions.

- Lithium toxicity occurs when sodium and fluid intake are insufficient, causing lithium retention.

- Amniotomy is the artificial rupture of the amniotic membranes.

- An alcoholic who achieves sobriety is called a *recovering alcoholic* because no cure for alcoholism exists.

- A patient is at greatest risk of dying during the first 24 to 48 hours after an MI.

- The left ventricle of the heart usually sustains the greatest damage during an MI.

- The pain of an MI results from myocardial ischemia caused by anoxia.

- For a patient in cardiac arrest, the first priority is to establish an airway.

- The universal sign for choking is clutching the hand to the throat.

- For a patient with congestive heart failure or cardiogenic pulmonary edema, nursing interventions focus on decreasing venous return to the heart and increasing left ventricular output; these interventions include placing the patient in a high-Fowler's position and administering oxygen, diuretics, and positive inotropic drugs as prescribed.

- A positive tuberculin skin test is an induration of 10 mm or more at the injection site.

- Histoplasmosis, a chronic systemic fungal infection, produces signs and symptoms that resemble those of tuberculosis (TB).

- Fluid oscillation in the tubing of a chest drainage system indicates that the system is working properly.

- In burn victims, the leading cause of death is respiratory compromise; the second leading cause is infection.

- The exocrine function of the pancreas is the secretion of enzymes used to digest carbohydrates, fats, and proteins.

- A patient with hepatitis A (infectious hepatitis) should consume a diet that is moderately high in fat and high in carbohydrate and protein and should eat the largest meal in the morning.

- The nurse should place a patient with a Sengstaken-Blakemore tube in the semi-Fowler's position.

- Esophageal varices can be visualized only by radiography (X-rays) or endoscopy.

- Prolactin overproduction by the pituitary gland can cause galactorrhea (excessive or abnormal lactation) and amenorrhea.

- A classic symptom of arterial insufficiency in the leg is intermittent claudication (pain during walking or other movement that is relieved with rest).

- During pregnancy, weight gain averages 25 to 30 lb (11.3 to 13.5 kg).

- In bladder carcinoma, the most common finding is gross, painless hematuria.

- The nurse can elicit Trousseau's sign by occluding the brachial or radial artery; hand and finger spasms during occlusion indicate Trousseau's sign and suggest hypocalcemia.

- The M'Naghten (McNaughten) rule is used as a criminal defense on grounds of insanity. It holds that at the time of the offense, the accused party was laboring under such a mental defect as not to know the quality and nature of the act.

- The Durham rule states that a person is not criminally responsible for committing an unlawful act if the act was a product of a mental disease or defect.

- According to Erikson, the school-age child (ages 6 to 12) is in the industry-versus-inferiority stage of psychosocial development.

- For a burn patient, care priorities include (1) maintaining a patent airway, (2) preventing or correcting fluid and electro-lyte imbalances, (3) controlling pain, and (4) preventing infection.

- Aspirin ingestion is the leading cause of poisoning in children.

- *Active immunization* refers to antibody formation within the body in response to vaccination or disease exposure.

- *Passive immunization* refers to administration of antibodies that were preformed outside the body.

- Chickenpox usually causes a rash that passes through four stages: macules, papules, vesicles, and crusts.

- Rubella has a teratogenic effect on the fetus during the first trimester and produces abnormalities in up to 40% of cases without interrupting the pregnancy.

- To calculate a pediatric dose using Clark's rule, the nurse should multiply the adult dose by the child's weight in pounds and divide the result by 150.

- To calculate a pediatric dose using Young's rule, the nurse should multiply the adult dose by the child's age in years and divide the result by the sum of the child's age plus 12.

- A patient receiving digoxin (Lanoxin) should not receive a calcium preparation because of the increased risk of digitalis toxicity. Concomitant use may affect cardiac contractility and lead to arrhythmias.

- For blood transfusion in an adult, the appropriate needle size is 18G or smaller.

- *Intermittent positive pressure breathing (IPPB)* refers to lung inflation (during inspiration) with compressed air or oxygen under pressure from a cycling valve.

- A laceration is a torn, jagged, or irregular wound.

- Wristdrop results from paralysis of the extensor muscles in the forearm and hand.

- Footdrop results from excessive plantar flexion and usually is a complication of prolonged bed rest.

- A patient with gonorrhea may be treated with penicillin and probenecid (Benemid). Probenecid delays penicillin excretion, keeping this antibiotic in the body longer.

- Pain that incapacitates a patient and cannot be relieved by drugs is called *intractable pain.*

- In an emergency, consent for treatment can be obtained by fax, telephone, or other telegraphic transmission.

- Decibel (dB) is the unit of measurement of sound.

- On-call medication is preanesthetic medication that should be ready for immediate administration when the call from surgery is received.

- If gagging, nausea, or vomiting occurs when an airway is removed, the nurse should place the patient in a lateral position with the upper arm supported on a pillow.

- Emancipated minors are individuals under the age of majority (usually age 18 or 21) who are not under parental control, such as married minors, those who serve in the military, and college students who live away from home.

- Informed consent is required for any invasive procedure.

- A patient who cannot write his or her name to give consent for treatment must have his or her X witnessed by two persons, such as a nurse, priest, or physician.

- When a postoperative patient arrives in the recovery room, the nurse should position the patient with the head turned to the side and the chin extended; Sims' position commonly is used.

- In the immediate postoperative period, the nurse should report a respiratory rate greater than 30, temperature over 100° F (37.5° C) or below 97° F (36.5° C), or a significant drop in blood pressure or rise in pulse rate from the baseline.

- Immunity to rubella can be measured by a hemagglutination inhibition test (rubella titre). This test identifies exposure to rubella infection and determines susceptibility to it in pregnant women.

- In describing the degree of fetal descent during labor, floating occurs when the presenting part is not engaged in the pelvic inlet but is freely movable (ballotable) above the pelvic inlet.

- If the central nervous system (CNS) is deprived of oxygen for more than 6 minutes, irreversible brain damage may occur.

- In describing the degree of fetal descent, engagement occurs when the largest diameter of the presenting part has passed through the pelvic inlet.

- The Z-track intramuscular (I.M.) injection technique seals medication deep into the muscle, thereby minimizing skin irritation and staining. It requires a needle that is 1" (2.5 cm) or longer.

- Fetal station (location of the presenting part) is described as –1, –2, –3, –4, or –5 to indicate the number of centimeters it is above the level of the ischial spines; station –5 is at the pelvic inlet.

- Fetal station also is described as +1, +2, +3, +4, or +5 to indicate the number of centimeters it is below the level of the ischial spines; station 0 is at the level of the ischial spines.

- During the first stage of labor, the side-lying position usually provides the greatest degree of comfort, although the patient may assume any position that is comfortable.

- During delivery, if umbilical cord loops cannot be loosened and slipped from around the neonate's neck, they should be clamped with two clamps and cut.

- The nurse assigns an Apgar score to a neonate at 1 and 5 minutes after delivery. A score of 7 to 10 indicates no immediate stress, 4 to 6 indicates moderate depression, and 0 to 3 indicates severe depression.

- A neonate born to a mother with gonorrhea should receive penicillin I.M.

- A patient with acute renal failure should receive a high-calorie diet that is low in protein and may be low in potassium and sodium.

- Addison's disease results from adrenal gland hypofunction and is characterized by fatigue, anemia, weight loss, and bronze skin pigmentation. It usually is fatal without cortisol replacement therapy.

- In the event of fire, the nurse should (1) remove the patient, (2) call the fire department, (3) attempt to contain the fire by closing the door, and (4) extinguish the fire, if it can be done safely.

- When caring for a depressed patient, the nurse's first priority is safety because of the increased risk of suicide.

- Glaucoma is managed conservatively with beta-adrenergic blockers, such as timolol (Timoptic), which decrease sympathetic impulses to the eye, and with miotic eyedrops, such as pilocarpine (Isopto Carpine), which constrict the pupils.

- Miotics effectively treat glaucoma by reducing intraocular pressure. They do this by constricting the pupil, contracting the ciliary muscles, opening the anterior chamber angle, and increasing the outflow of aqueous humor.

- While a patient is receiving heparin, the nurse should monitor the partial thromboplastin time (PTT).

- Urinary frequency, incontinence, or both can occur after catheter removal. Incontinence may be manifested as dribbling.

- When teaching a patient about colostomy care, the nurse should instruct the patient to hang the irrigation reservoir 18" to 22" (45 to 55 cm) above the stoma, irrigate the stoma once a day, clean the area around the stoma with soap and water before applying a new bag, and use a protective skin covering, such as a Stomahesive wafer, karaya paste, or karaya ring, around the stoma.

- Two hours after eating, a patient with a duodenal ulcer is most likely to report pain, which can be relieved by eating food, drinking milk, or taking an antacid.

- A registered nurse (RN) should assign a licensed vocational nurse (LVN) or licensed practical nurse (LPN) to perform bedside care, such as suctioning and medication administration.

- Continuous bubbling in a one-bottle water-seal chest drainage system indicates that air is leaking into the system.

- During or shortly after eating, a patient with a gastric ulcer is most likely to report pain.

- A sign of increasing intracranial pressure is widening pulse pressure. For example, the blood pressure may rise from 120/80 to 160/60 mm Hg.

- In a burn victim, a primary goal of wound care is to prevent contamination by microorganisms.

- To prevent external rotation in a patient who has had hip nailing, the nurse places trochanter rolls from the knee to the ankle of the affected leg.

- Severe hip pain after the insertion of a hip prosthesis indicates dislodgment. If this occurs, the nurse should assess the leg and then call the physician.

- To elicit Moro's reflex, the nurse should hold the neonate in both hands and suddenly but gently drop the neonate's head backward. Normally, this causes the neonate to abduct and extend all extremities bilaterally and symmetrically, form a C shape with thumb and forefinger, and first adduct and then flex the extremities.

- Echolalia is the parrot-like repetition of another person's words or phrases. It commonly occurs in schizophrenia.

- According to psychoanalytic theory, the ego is the part of the psyche that controls internal demands and interacts with the outside world at the conscious, preconscious, and unconscious levels.

• According to psychoanalytic theory, the superego is the part of the psyche that is composed of morals, values, and ethics. It is the aspect that continually evaluates thoughts and actions, rewarding the good and punishing the bad. (Think of the superego as the "supercop" of the unconscious.)

• According to psychoanalytic theory, the id is the part of the psyche that contains instinctual drives. (Remember *i* for instinctual and *d* for drive.)

• According to Erikson, the child from birth to age 18 months is in the trust-versus-mistrust stage of psychosocial development.

• Pregnancy-induced hypertension (preeclampsia) is defined as an increase in blood pressure of 30/15 mm Hg over baseline or 140/95 mm Hg on two occasions at least 6 hours apart, edema, and albuminuria that occur after 20 weeks' gestation.

• Positive signs and symptoms of pregnancy include ultrasound evidence, fetal heart tones, and fetal movement felt by the examiner (not usually present until 4 months' gestation).

• Goodell's sign is softening of the cervix.

• Hegar's sign is softening of the lower uterine segment.

• Quickening, a presumptive sign of pregnancy, occurs between 16 and 19 weeks' gestation.

• Ovulation ceases during pregnancy.

• Vaginal bleeding is the number one danger sign during pregnancy.

• To estimate the date of confinement using Nagle's rule, the nurse counts backward 3 months from the first day of the last menstrual period and then adds 7 days to this date.

- At 12 weeks' gestation, the fundus should be at the top of the symphysis pubis.

- Koplik's spots are small, irregular red spots with minute bluish white centers that appear on the buccal mucosa of patients with measles (rubeola).

- Up to 75% of renal function must be lost before blood urea nitrogen (BUN) and serum creatinine levels rise above normal.

- The nephrons filter 125 ml of blood per minute.

- *Polyuria* refers to a urine output of 2,000 ml or more within 8 hours.

- The therapeutic purpose of a mist tent is to increase hydration of secretions.

- Pancreatin replacement therapy is used to promote protein absorption.

- In a patient who cannot void, the first nursing action should be assessment by bladder palpation.

- If a patient has a gastric drainage tube in place, the nurse should expect the physician to order potassium chloride.

- Cow's milk should not be given to infants under age 1 year because of its low linoleic acid content and its protein, which is difficult for infants to digest.

- An increased pulse rate is one of the first indications of respiratory difficulty. It occurs because the heart attempts to compensate for a decreased oxygen supply to the tissues by pumping more blood.

- If physiologic jaundice is suspected, the nurse should examine the infant under natural light from a window. If unavailable, the nurse should examine the infant under a white light.

• Denial is the defense mechanism used by a patient who denies the reality of an event.

• To remember the action of the diuretic furosemide (Lasix), keep in mind that it *la*sts for *six* hours.

• The patient who uses a cane should carry it on the unaffected side.

• The patient with leg injury should advance the unaffected side first when climbing stairs and advance the affected leg first when descending stairs.

• To fit a supine patient for crutches, the nurse should measure from the axilla to the sole and add 2" (5 cm).

• A labor contraction's intensity can be assessed by the indentability of the uterine wall at the contraction's peak. Intensity is graded as mild (uterine muscle is somewhat tense), moderate (uterine muscle is moderately tense), or strong (uterine muscle is board-like).

• *Chloasma*, the mask of pregnancy, refers to skin pigmentation of a circumscribed area (usually over the bridge of the nose and cheeks), which may occur during pregnancy.

• The gynecoid pelvis is most ideal for delivery. Other types include platypelloid, anthropoid, and android.

• Pregnant women should be advised that there is no safe level of alcohol intake.

• In an adult, a hemoglobin level below 11 mg/dl indicates iron deficiency anemia.

• The normal partial pressure of oxygen (PaO_2) in arterial blood is 95 mm Hg (plus or minus 5 mm Hg).

• Vitamin C deficiency is characterized by brittle bones, pinpoint peripheral hemorrhages, and friable gums with loosened teeth.

- Functional nursing uses the task-oriented approach in which the nurse focuses on specific jobs that need to be accomplished, such as treatments.

- In a psychiatric setting, seclusion is used to promote therapeutic limit-setting, reduce overwhelming environmental stimulation, protect the patient from self-injury or injury to others, and prevent damage to hospital property. It is used for patients who do not respond to less restrictive interventions and controls external behavior until the patient can assume self-control and supports the patient in regaining self-control.

- In a patient who takes a monoamine oxidase (MAO) inhibitor, severe hypertension may occur if the patient eats tyramine-rich food, such as aged cheese, chicken liver, avocados, bananas, meat tenderizer, salami, bologna, Chianti wine, and beer.

- A patient who takes an MAO inhibitor should be weighed biweekly and monitored for suicidal tendencies. If palpitations, headaches, or severe orthostatic hypotension occurs, the nurse should withhold medication and notify the physician.

- Normally, intraocular pressure ranges from 12 to 20 mm Hg. It is measured with a Schiøtz's tonometer.

- A contraction's frequency is measured in minutes and represents the time from the beginning of one contraction to the beginning of the next.

- In early hemorrhagic shock, the patient's blood pressure may be normal, but the respiratory and pulse rates are rapid. The patient may complain of thirst, have clammy skin, and develop piloerection (goose bumps).

- Assessment begins with the nurse's first encounter with the patient and continues throughout the patient's stay. The nurse obtains assessment data through the health history, physical examination, and review of diagnostic studies.

• Cool, moist, pale skin—as occurs in shock—results from diversion of blood from the skin to the major organs.

• To assess capillary refill, the nurse applies pressure over the nail bed until blanching occurs, quickly releases the pressure, and notes the rate at which blanching fades. Capillary refill assesses perfusion, which decreases in shock, thereby lengthening the refill time.

• Except for patients with renal failure, low urine output signifies dehydration and the potential for shock.

• The nursing process is a systematic, problem-solving method of providing nursing care.

• The appropriate needle size for an insulin injection is 25G and 5/8" (1.5 cm) long.

• Residual urine is urine that remains in the bladder after voiding. The amount of residual urine normally ranges from 50 to 100 ml.

• The most common fracture in elderly patients is hip fracture. Osteoporosis weakens the bones, predisposing these patients to fracture, which usually results from a fall.

• The five stages of the nursing process are assessment, nursing diagnosis, planning, implementation, and evaluation.

• Planning is the stage of the nursing process in which the nurse assigns priorities to nursing diagnoses, defines short-term and long-term goals and expected outcomes, and establishes the nursing care plan.

• Implementation is the stage of the nursing process in which the nurse puts the nursing care plan into action, delegates specific nursing interventions to members of the nursing team, and charts patient responses to nursing interventions.

- Evaluation is the stage of the nursing process in which the nurse compares objective and subjective data with the outcome criteria and, if needed, modifies the nursing care plan, making the nursing process circular.

- The acronym *SOAP* represents a format used to write nursing progress notes: The S stands for subjective data, O for objective data, A for assessment, and P for plan.

- In the SOAP format, subjective data are provided by the patient and cover the time period since the last entry in the health record.

- In the SOAP format, objective data consists of information that can be observed or measured and include physical examination findings and the results of laboratory tests and other diagnostic studies.

- In the SOAP format, assessment is an evaluation of subjective (S) and objective (O) data as well as the cause of the problem, course of the disease, and patient's response to therapy. It includes a statement of the patient's participation in the nursing care plan and the patient's reaction to treatment.

- In the SOAP format, the plan specifies what must be done, who must do it, and when it must be done.

- The level of amputation is determined by estimating the maximum viable tissue (tissue with adequate circulation) needed to develop a functional stump.

- Before internal fetal monitoring can be done, a pregnant patient's cervix must be dilated at least 2 cm, her amniotic membranes must be ruptured, and the fetus's presenting part (scalp or buttocks) must be at station −1 or lower, so that a small electrode can be clipped to it.

- Fetal alcohol syndrome occurs in the first 24 hours after birth and produces lethargy, seizures, poor sucking reflex, abdominal distention, and respiratory difficulty.

- *Variability* refers to any change in the fetal heart rate (FHR) from its normal rate of 120 to 160 beats/minute. An increased FHR is known as *acceleration*; a decreased FHR is known as *deceleration.*

- Hexachlorophene (pHisoHex) no longer is used to bathe infants because it may cause neurotoxicity.

- Heroin withdrawal symptoms in a neonate may begin several hours to 4 days after birth.

- Methadone withdrawal symptoms in a neonate may begin 7 days to several weeks after birth.

- The cardinal signs of neonatal narcotic withdrawal include coarse flapping tremors, sleepiness, restlessness, prolonged and persistent high-pitched cry, and irritability.

- The nurse should count an infant's respirations for 1 full minute.

- Paroxysmal nocturnal dyspnea may indicate congestive heart failure.

- For a patient who takes a digitalis compound, such as digoxin or digitoxin, the diet should include high-potassium foods.

- The nurse should limit tracheobronchial suctioning to 10 to 15 seconds. Suctioning should never exceed 15 seconds.

- Before performing tracheobronchial suctioning, the nurse should ventilate and oxygenate the patient five to six times with a resuscitation bag and 100% oxygen. This procedure is called *bagging.*

- Signs and symptoms of pneumothorax include tachypnea, restlessness, and hypotension.

- The first cardinal sign of toxic shock syndrome is rapid onset of a high fever.

- A key sign of peptic ulcer is hematemesis, which can be bright red or dark red with the consistency of coffee grounds.

- Signs and symptoms of a perforated peptic ulcer include sudden, severe upper abdominal pain, vomiting, and an extremely tender and rigid (board-like) abdomen.

- Constipation is a common adverse reaction to aluminum hydroxide.

- For the first few days after an MI, a patient should use a bedside commode.

- Circumcision is postponed in neonates with hypospadias.

- Activity that requires heavy exertion is prohibited for at least 6 months in a patient who has had an MI.

- In a patient who recently has had an MI, frothy, blood-tinged sputum suggests pulmonary edema.

- The primary purpose of drugs prescribed for a patient with acquired immunodeficiency syndrome (AIDS) is to prevent secondary infections.

- Immune system suppression places a patient with AIDS at risk for developing opportunistic infections, such as *Pneumocystis carinii* pneumonia, and thrush.

- A patient with AIDS may experience rapid weight loss, which is known as *wasting syndrome.*

- Between ages 10 and 12 months, a child begins to show emotions, such as affection, jealousy, and anger.

- Chlorpromazine hydrochloride (Thorazine) is used to treat an infant who is addicted to narcotics.

- The nurse should use elbow restraints for protection on an infant with eczema or a scalp vein infusion or one who is recovering from cleft lip repair or eye surgery.

• The nurse should provide a dark, quiet environment for an infant who is experiencing narcotic withdrawal.

• A good technique for assessing jaundice in a neonate is to blanch the tip of the nose or gum line by applying slight pressure under natural light and watching for yellow discoloration after removing pressure.

• The normal fasting blood glucose level in children is 60 to 100 mg/ml of blood.

• If the body does not use glucose for energy, it metabolizes fat for energy, which results in ketone production.

• Separation from the mother evokes the most intense response in infants from age 6 to 12 months.

• Because steroids mask symptoms of infection, they should be administered to children with extreme caution.

• Steroids should be administered to a child with food.

• Leukemia is the most common cancer during childhood.

• Signs and symptoms of leukemia in children include fatigue, anorexia, low-grade fever, and decreased white blood cell (WBC), red blood cell (RBC), and platelet counts.

• In a child with leukemia, the most common cause of death is hemorrhage or infection.

• Anemia is the first sign of lead poisoning in a child.

• The nurse should place a child with a spica cast in the prone or supine position. A Bradford frame often is used for immobilization.

• The first sign of respiratory distress in a premature infant is nostril flaring.

• The first emotional response in an infant is the need for affection.

- Having and frequently speaking to an imaginary friend are normal behaviors in a child age 3.

- An infant with normal motor development should be able to lift and control the head (replace head lag) by age 3 to 4 months.

- Thrush is candidiasis (*Candida albicans*) of the oral mucous membranes. It is characterized by aphthae, or small ulcers, in the mouth.

- A common cause of child abuse is poor impulse control by parents.

- Allopurinol (Zyloprim) is used in pediatric patients with leukemia to prevent uric acid accumulation.

- Before administering any p.r.n. pain medication, the nurse should ask the patient to indicate the pain's location.

- At age 6 months, an infant should begin to receive solid foods one at a time and 1 week apart.

- After percutaneous bladder aspiration, the patient's first void normally may be pink. However, urine with frank blood should be reported to the physician.

- The American Academy of Pediatrics recommends that an infant's first immunizations should be for diphtheria, pertussis, and tetanus (DPT) and for polio.

- The most appropriate toy for a toddler age 18 months is one that helps develop motor coordination.

- When administering an injection to an infant, the nurse should ask another nurse to divert the child's attention and assist as needed.

- Premature infants develop respiratory distress syndrome (RDS, or hyaline membrane disease) because their pulmonary alveoli lack surfactant.

- After breast-feeding, the mother should position the infant on the side.

✓ • A patient undergoing dialysis should take a vitamin supplement and eat foods that are high in calories but low in protein, sodium, and potassium.

- The nurse should not give anything by mouth to a patient who is experiencing dyspnea.

- For an infant with phenylketonuria, the nurse should provide a low-phenylalanine formula and monitor plasma phenylalanine levels frequently.

- When caring for an infant who has had diarrhea six to eight times a day for 4 days, the nurse should assess for electrolyte imbalance.

- The nurse may offer finger foods to a child age 3 who has a poor appetite.

- When in a mist tent (Croupette), a child may require soft restraints.

- In a patient with chronic obstructive pulmonary disease (COPD), the most effective way to reduce thick secretions is by forcing fluids.

- The nurse should not administer medication to a child at bedtime unless specifically prescribed because it may stimulate the child.

- Medulloblastoma, the most common brain tumor in children, characteristically is found in the cerebellum.

- The nurse should teach a patient with emphysema how to perform pursed-lip breathing because it slows expiration, prevents alveolar collapse, and helps control the respiratory rate.

- A patient with COPD may develop finger clubbing.

- A cerebrovascular accident (CVA), or stroke, disrupts the brain's blood supply and may be caused by hypertension.

- Aminophylline (Aminophyllin) and theophylline (Theo-Dur) are bronchodilators.

- Chest percussion therapy helps loosen bronchial secretions.

- The most reliable and accurate way to administer oxygen to a patient with COPD is by a Venturi mask.

- Isoetharine hydrochloride (Bronkosol) can be administered by a hand-held nebulizer or IPPB.

- Brain death is the irreversible cessation of brain function.

- Skin-fold measurements are used to evaluate subcutaneous fat stores.

- The classic adverse reactions to antihistamines are dry mouth, drowsiness, and blurred vision.

- A patient who has received a general anesthetic cannot take anything by mouth until active bowel sounds are heard in all abdominal quadrants.

- Jehovah's Witnesses believe that they should not receive blood components donated by other people.

- A patient with diabetic ketoacidosis (DKA) is a great risk of developing shock.

- A patient with diabetes is susceptible to atherosclerosis, which can cause intermittent claudication.

- Cough medications that contain codeine help suppress the cough reflex.

- Before removing a foreign body from a patient's eye, the nurse should check the patient's visual acuity.

• When phenylephrine hydrochloride (Neo-Synephrine) is instilled in a patient's eye, mydriasis should occur.

• To test visual acuity, the nurse should ask the patient to cover each eye separately and read the eye chart with glasses and without, as appropriate.

• A cataract is an opacity of the crystalline lens.

• To assess a corneal abrasion, fluorescein staining commonly is used because it outlines superficial epithelial defects.

• Presbyopia (far-sightedness) typically is caused by old age.

• When providing oral care for an unconscious patient, the nurse should position the patient on the side to minimize the risk of aspiration.

• During assessment of distance vision, the patient should stand 20 ft (6.1 m) from the chart.

• Transient ischemic attacks are warning signs of an impending CVA.

• A sign of acute appendicitis, McBurney's sign is tenderness at McBurney's point (about 2" [5 cm] from the right anterior superior iliac spine on a line between the spine and the umbilicus).

• When caring for a patient with Guillain-Barré syndrome, the nurse should focus on respiratory interventions.

• The diagnosis of Alzheimer's disease is based on clinical findings of two or more cognitive deficits, progressive worsening of memory, and the results of a neuropsychological test.

• Signs and symptoms of colon cancer include rectal bleeding, change in bowel habits, intestinal obstruction, abdominal pain, weight loss, anorexia, nausea, and vomiting.

- Memory disturbance is a classic sign of Alzheimer's disease.

- To help calm a child who is frightened of a mist tent, the nurse may suggest that a parent lie with the child in the tent.

- The tonsils and adenoids help defend the body against respiratory infections.

- The male sperm may contribute an X or a Y chromosome; the female ovum contributes an X chromosome.

- Fertilization produces a total of 46 chromosomes, including an XY combination (male) or an XX combination (female).

 • A chancre is a painless, ulcerative lesion that develops during the primary stage of syphilis.

- During the tertiary stage of syphilis, spirochetes invade the internal organs and cause permanent damage.

- The ideal room temperature for a geriatric patient or one who is extremely ill ranges from 66° to 76° F (18.8° to 24.4° C).

- Normal room humidity ranges from 30% to 60%.

- Hand washing is the single best method of limiting the spread of microorganisms.

- The percentage of water in an infant's body is about 78% to 80%.

- In total parenteral nutrition (TPN), weight gain is the most reliable indicator of a positive response to therapy.

- The nurse may administer an intravenous (I.V.) fat emulsion through a central or peripheral catheter but should not use an in-line filter because the fat particles are too large to pass through the pores.

- To catheterize a female patient, the nurse should place her in the dorsal recumbent position.

- A positive Homan's sign may indicate thrombophlebitis.

- Electrolytes in a solution are measured in milliequivalents per liter (mEq/L).

- An elixir is a liquid that contains alcohol, sugar, or a flavoring substance and primarily is used as a vehicle for an oral drug.

- Thought blocking is the loss of the train of thought because of a mental defect.

- A Bradford frame is used for a child who must be immobilized for a long period, such as one with extensive burns or meningocele or one who has a spica cast.

- Metabolism takes place in two phases: anabolism (the constructive phase) and catabolism (the destructive phase).

- In anabolism, larger molecules are made from smaller ones to promote growth and repair.

- In catabolism, larger molecules are broken down to smaller ones to produce fuel for the body.

- The basal metabolic rate (BMR) represents the amount of energy needed to maintain essential body functions. It is measured when the patient is awake and resting, has not eaten for 14 to 18 hours, and is in a comfortable, warm environment.

- The BMR is expressed in calories consumed per hour per kilogram of body weight.

- Cheilosis produces fissures at the angles of the mouth and indicates a vitamin B_2 or riboflavin deficiency.

- Tetany may result from hypocalcemia.

• Dietary fiber (roughage), which is derived from cellulose, supplies bulk, maintains adequate intestinal motility, and helps establish regular bowel habits.

• Alcohol is metabolized primarily in the liver. Smaller amounts are metabolized by the kidneys and lungs.

• Proteins are the major source of building material for muscles, blood, skin, hair, nails, and internal organs.

• Commonly caused by cirrhosis, ascites is the accumulation of fluid (that contains large amounts of protein and electrolytes) in the abdominal cavity.

• The nurse may assess obesity by measuring the patient's skin-fold thickness, which reflects subcutaneous adipose tissue.

• RBCs transport hemoglobin, WBCs fight infection, and platelets promote coagulation.

• Hemophilia is a bleeding disorder that is transmitted genetically in a sex-linked (X chromosome) recessive pattern. Although women carry the defective gene, only men develop the disorder.

• Von Willebrand's disease is an autosomal dominant bleeding disorder that results from platelet dysfunction and Factor VIII deficiency.

• Sickle cell anemia, a congenital hemolytic anemia, is caused by defective hemoglobin S molecules and primarily affects black patients.

• Sickle cell anemia results from homozygous inheritance; sickle cell trait results from heterozygous inheritance.

• A characteristic sign of Hodgkin's disease, Pel-Ebstein fever recurs every few days or weeks and alternates with afebrile periods.

- Petechiae are tiny, round purplish red spots that appear on the skin and mucous membranes as a result of intradermal or submucosal hemorrhage.

- *Purpura* refers to any purple skin discoloration caused by blood extravasation.

- Glucose-6-phosphate dehydrogenase (G6PD) deficiency is an inherited metabolic disorder characterized by RBCs that are deficient in G6PD, a critical enzyme in aerobic glycolysis.

- Preferred sites for bone marrow aspiration are the posterior superior iliac crest, anterior iliac crest, and sternum.

- During bone marrow harvesting, the donor receives general anesthesia and 400 to 800 ml of marrow are aspirated.

- A butterfly rash across the bridge of the nose is a characteristic sign of systemic lupus erythematosus (SLE).

- Rheumatoid arthritis is a chronic, destructive collagen disease characterized by symmetric inflammation of the synovium, which leads to joint swelling.

- A compulsion is an irresistible urge to perform an irrational act, such as walking in a clockwise circle before leaving a room.

- A patient with a chosen method and a plan to commit suicide in the next 48 to 72 hours is at high risk for suicide.

- Screening for human immunodeficiency virus (HIV) antibodies begins with the enzyme-linked immunosorbent assay (ELISA) and is confirmed by the Western blot test.

- The therapeutic serum level for lithium is 0.5 to 1.5 mEq/liter.

- Desensitization therapy, which gradually exposes a patient to a stimulus, is used to treat phobic disorders.

- Dysfunctional grieving is grief that is prolonged beyond the usual time.

- To perform nasotracheal suctioning in an infant, the nurse should position the infant with the neck slightly hyperextended in a "sniffing" position with the chin up and the head tilted back slightly.

- The nurse should suction an infant quickly and gently to avoid hypoxia and apnea. (More prolonged suctioning may be used if the nurse administers oxygen by hand-held resuscitation bag between suctioning periods.)

- Organogenesis occurs during the first trimester of pregnancy.

- After birth, the neonate's umbilical cord is tied 1" (2.5 cm) from the abdominal wall with a cotton cord, plastic clamp, or rubber band.

- The term -*gravida* refers to the number of pregnancies regardless of their outcomes.

- The term -*para* refers to the number of viable young, regardless of whether the births were live or stillborn.

- An ectopic pregnancy is one that implants abnormally, outside the uterus.

- The first stage of labor begins with the onset of labor and ends with full cervical dilation at 10 cm (4").

- The second stage of labor begins with full cervical dilation and ends with the neonate's birth.

- The third stage of labor begins after the neonate's birth and ends with expulsion of the placenta.

- In a full-term infant, deep skin creases appear over the entire sole; in a preterm infant, deep creases appear only on the anterior third of the foot.

- The fourth stage of labor (postpartal stabilization) lasts for up to 4 hours after delivery of the placenta (the time required to stabilize the mother's physical and emotional state after the stress of childbirth).

- At 20 weeks' gestation, the fundus should be at the height of the umbilicus.

- At 36 weeks' gestation, the fundus should be at 1the lower border of the rib cage.

- A premature infant is one born before the end of the 37th week of gestation.

- Developmental disorders of the phallic stage are transsexuality and preoccupation with sexual attractiveness.

- During phase I of the nurse-patient relationship (beginning or orientation phase), an initial history is obtained and a mutual contract is agreed on.

- During phase II of the nurse-patient relationship (middle or working phase), the patient discusses problems, behavioral changes occur, and self-defeating behavior is resolved or reduced.

- During phase III of the nurse-patient relationship (termination or resolution phase), the nurse terminates the therapeutic relationship and gives the patient positive feedback on accomplishments.

- Pregnancy-induced hypertension is a leading cause of maternal death in the United States.

- A habitual abortionist is a woman who has had three or more spontaneous abortions.

- Threatened abortion occurs when bleeding is present without cervical dilation.

- A complete abortion occurs when all products of conception have been expelled.

- Hydramnios (polyhydramnios) is excessive amniotic fluid (more than 2,000 ml in the third trimester).

- Excessive vitamin K intake may significantly antagonize the anticoagulant effects of warfarin (Coumadin).

- According to the universal precautions recommended by the Centers for Disease Control and Prevention (CDCP), the nurse should not recap needles after use because most needlesticks result from missed needle recapping.

- According to Freud, a person between ages 12 and 20 is in the genital stage, during which he or she learns independence, has increased interest in members of the opposite sex, and establishes an identity.

- According to Erikson, the identity-versus-role confusion stage occurs between ages 12 and 20.

- A person who has been involuntarily admitted to a mental health unit may request freedom by obtaining a writ of *habeas corpus* (a court petition that protects against illegal imprisonment).

- Tolerance is the need for increasing amounts of a substance to achieve an effect that formerly was achieved with lesser amounts.

- The antidote for heparin overdose is protamine sulfate.

- A lymph node biopsy that shows Reed-Sternberg cells provides a definitive diagnosis of Hodgkin's disease.

- The nurse should remove a child's mitts twice each shift to let the child exercise the fingers.

- Stress, dehydration, and fatigue may reduce a breast-feeding mother's milk supply.

- Bell's palsy is unilateral facial weakness or paralysis caused by a disturbance of the seventh cranial (facial) nerve.

- During the transition phase of the first stage of labor, the cervix is dilated 7 to 10 cm and contractions usually occur 2 to 3 minutes apart and last for 60 seconds.

- A nonstress test is considered nonreactive (positive) if fewer than two FHR accelerations of at least 15 beats/minute occur in 20 minutes.

- A nonstress test is considered reactive (negative) if two or more FHR accelerations of 15 beats/minute above baseline occur in 20 minutes.

- A nonstress test usually is used to assess fetal well-being in a pregnant patient with a prolonged pregnancy (42 weeks or more), diabetes, a history of poor pregnancy outcomes, or pregnancy-induced hypertension.

- The nurse administers a drug by I.V. push by delivering the dose directly into a vein, I.V. tubing, or cannula with a needle and syringe.

- When feeding an infant through a tracheostomy tube, the nurse should cover the tube opening with moistened gauze. (A bib may be used for a child over age 1.)

- When changing the ties on a tracheostomy tube, the nurse should leave the old ties in place until the new ones are applied.

- A nurse always should have assistance when changing the ties on a tracheostomy tube.

- The nurse should not lift an infant by the legs to change a diaper.

- To prevent urine from running under a spica cast, the nurse should elevate the head of the patient's bed higher than the foot of the bed.

- A spica cast dries completely in 24 to 48 hours.

- During an initial tuberculin skin test, lack of a wheal after injection of tuberculin purified protein derivative indicates that the test dose was injected too deeply and that the nurse should inject another dose at least 2" (5 cm) from the initial site.

- A tuberculin skin test should be read 48 to 72 hours after administration.

- In response to a tuberculin skin test, erythema without induration is not significant.

- Death from botulism usually results from delayed diagnosis and respiratory complications.

- In a patient with rabies, saliva contains the rabies virus and constitutes a hazard for nurses who provide care.

- A pregnant woman should drink at least eight 8-oz glasses (about 2,000 ml) of water daily.

- Usually, the nurse uses a 170-micron in-line filter for blood transfusions.

- The most common transfusion reaction is a febrile non-hemolytic reaction.

- A four-point (quad) cane is indicated when a patient needs more stability than a regular cane can provide.

- The patient should carry a cane on the unaffected side to promote a reciprocal gait pattern and distribute weight away from the affected leg.

- A good way to begin a patient interview is to ask "What made you seek medical help?"

- The nurse should adhere to universal precautions for blood and body fluids when caring for all patients.

- Potassium (K+) is the most abundant cation in intracellular fluid.

- Hypokalemia (abnormally low potassium concentration in the blood) may cause muscle weakness or paralysis, electrocardiographic (ECG) abnormalities, and GI disturbances.

- In the four-point gait (or alternating gait), the patient first moves the right crutch followed by the left foot and then the left crutch followed by the right foot.

- In the three-point gait, the patient moves two crutches and the affected leg simultaneously and then moves the unaffected leg.

- In the two-point gait, the patient moves the right leg and the left crutch simultaneously and then moves the left leg and the right crutch.

- Vitamin B complex, the water-soluble vitamins essential for metabolism, include thiamine (B_1), riboflavin (B_2), niacin (B_3), pyridoxine (B_6), and cyanocobalamin (B_{12}).

- When being weighed, an adult patient should be lightly dressed and shoeless.

- Beriberi, a serious vitamin B_1 (thiamine) deficiency, is epidemic in Asian countries where people subsist on unenriched rice and also affects alcoholics with poor dietary habits. It is characterized by the phrase "I cannot," indicating that the affected patient is too ill to do anything.

- Before taking an adult's oral temperature, the nurse should ensure that the patient has not smoked or consumed hot or cold substances in the past 15 minutes.

- The nurse should not take a rectal temperature if the patient has a cardiac disorder, anal lesions, or bleeding hemorrhoids or has recently undergone rectal surgery.

- Excessive sedation may cause respiratory depression.

- In a patient with cardiac problems, rectal temperature measurement may stimulate a vagal response, leading to vasodilation and decreased cardiac output.

- When recording pulse amplitude and rhythm, the nurse should use these descriptive measures: +3 indicates a bounding pulse (readily palpable and forceful); +2, a normal pulse (easily palpable); +1, a thready or weak pulse (difficult to detect); and 0, an absent pulse (not detectable).

- A preoperative method of teaching a child about postoperative events is to describe them using a life-size doll that has an incision, a dressing, a cast, or an I.V. line, as appropriate.

- The intraoperative period begins when a patient is transferred to the operating room bed and ends when the patient is admitted to the postanesthesia recovery unit.

- On the morning of surgery, the nurse should ensure that the informed consent form has been signed; that the patient has not taken anything by mouth since midnight, has taken a shower with antimicrobial soap, has had mouth care (without swallowing the water), has removed common jewelry, and has received preoperative medication as prescribed; and that vital signs have been taken and recorded.

- The primary postoperative concern is maintenance of a patent airway.

- If cyanosis occurs circumorally, sublingually, or in the nail bed, the oxygen saturation level is below 80%.

- A rapid pulse rate in a postoperative patient may indicate pain, bleeding, dehydration, or shock.

- Increased pulse rate and blood pressure may indicate that a patient is experiencing "silent pain" (pain that cannot be expressed verbally, such as when a patient is recovering from anesthesia).

• The postoperative systolic blood pressure reading should not be more than 50% higher than the preoperative baseline measurement.

• Cullen's sign (a bluish discoloration around the umbilicus of a postoperative patient) signals intra-abdominal or peritoneal bleeding.

• Comfort measures, such as positioning the patient, performing backrubs, and providing a restful environment, may decrease the patient's need for analgesics or may enhance their effectiveness.

• During the postoperative period, the patient should cough and deep breathe every 2 hours.

• Before surgery, a patient's respiratory volume may be measured by incentive spirometry. This measurement becomes the patient's postoperative goal for respiratory volume.

• The postoperative patient should use incentive spirometry 10 to 12 times per hour and take deep inhalations.

• Before ambulating, a postoperative patient should dangle the legs over the side of the bed and perform deep-breathing exercises.

• During the patient's first postoperative ambulation, the nurse should monitor closely and assist as needed while the patient walks a few feet from the bed to a steady chair.

• Hypovolemia occurs when 15% to 25% of the body's total blood volume is lost.

• Signs and symptoms of hypovolemia include rapid, weak pulse; low blood pressure; cool, clammy skin; shallow respirations; oliguria or anuria; and lethargy.

• In postoperative patients, the organism most likely to cause septicemia is *Escherichia coli.*

- Signs and symptoms of septicemia include fever, chills, rash, abdominal distention, prostration, pain, headache, nausea, and diarrhea.

- Rocky Mountain spotted fever can result from the bite of an infected wood tick or dog tick and produces a persistent high fever, nonpitting edema, and rash.

- A common sign of pernicious anemia is a red, beefy tongue.

- After routine patient contact, hand washing for 30 seconds usually is sufficient to reduce the spread of organisms.

- When both breasts are used for breast-feeding, the infant usually does not empty the second breast. This breast should be used first in the next feeding.

- After feeding an infant, the care giver should place the infant on the side to prevent aspiration.

- The patient should not void for 1 hour before percutaneous suprapubic bladder aspiration to ensure that sufficient urine remains in the bladder to make the procedure successful.

- Left-sided heart failure is manifested in pulmonary congestion, pink-tinged sputum, and dyspnea. (Think of L for *l*eft and *l*ung.)

- When applying a rubber band tourniquet on an infant's head, the nurse should place a second rubber band crosswise under it to facilitate lifting and cutting the tourniquet when it is removed.

- A low-birth-weight (LBW) infant is one who weighs 1,500 to 2,500 g (3 lb 5 oz to 5 lb 8 oz) at birth, regardless of gestational age.

- A very-low-birth-weight infant is one who weighs less than 1,500 g at birth.

• When lifting an infant, the nurse should maintain two points of contact with the infant's body at all times.

• When teaching parents to provide umbilical cord care, the nurse should teach them to wipe the umbilical area with alcohol on a cotton ball after every diaper change to prevent infection and promote drying.

• Parents of young children should set their water heater thermostat no higher than 130° F (54° C).

• Suicide is the third leading cause of death among teenagers.

• Most teenagers who kill themselves had made a previous suicide attempt and had left telltale signs of their plans.

• The nurse should teach a teenage girl that the most effective birth control method is abstinence and the second most effective method is oral contraceptive use.

• Teenage mothers are more likely to have LBW infants because they seek prenatal care late in their pregnancies (as a result of denial) and are more likely to have nutritional deficiencies.

• When obtaining a blood sample for arterial blood gas (ABG) analysis, the nurse should check the patient's collateral blood supply with the Allen's test *before* taking blood from a radial artery.

• When caring for a patient who is having a seizure, the nurse should follow these guidelines: (1) Avoid restraining the patient, but help a standing patient to a lying position. (2) Loosen restrictive clothing. (3) Place a pillow or other soft material under the patient's head. (4) Clear the area of hard objects. (5) Do not force anything into the patient's mouth, but maintain a patent airway. (6) Reassure and reorient the patient after the seizure subsides.

- An adverse reaction to phenytoin (Dilantin) is gingival hyperplasia.

- A drug has three names: its generic name, which is used in official publications; its trade name or brand name (such as Tylenol), which is selected by the drug company; and its chemical name, which describes the drug's chemical composition.

- The patient should take a liquid iron preparation through a straw to avoid staining the teeth.

- The nurse should use the Z-track method to administer an I.M. injection of iron dextran (Imferon).

- An organism may enter the body through the nose, mouth, rectum, urinary or reproductive tract, or skin.

- According to Maslow's hierarchy of needs, physiologic needs must be satisfied before other needs can be addressed.

- Love and belonging needs consist of affiliation, affection, and intimacy.

- Self-esteem needs consist of feelings of self-worth, self-respect, independence, self-reliance, and dignity.

- Self-actualization needs consist of recognition and use of one's unique potential and abilities.

- Linea nigra, a dark line that extends from the umbilicus to the mons pubis, commonly appears during pregnancy.

- Implantation in the uterus occurs 6 to 10 days after ovum fertilization.

- In Erikson's stage of generativity versus despair, generativity (investment of self in the interest of the larger community) is expressed through procreation as well as through work, community service, and creative endeavors.

- Most infants double their birth weight by age 5 to 6 months and triple it by age 1 year.

- For the first 24 hours after amputation, the nurse should elevate the patient's stump to prevent edema.

- Lung cancer is the most common cancer among men.

- In descending order, the levels of consciousness are alertness, lethargy, stupor, light coma, and deep coma.

- Parkinson's disease characteristically produces progressive muscle rigidity, akinesia, and involuntary tremor.

- Tonic-clonic (grand mal) seizures are characterized by a loss of consciousness and alternating periods of muscle contraction and relaxation.

- Status epilepticus, a life-threatening emergency, is a series of rapidly repeating seizures without intervening periods of consciousness.

- The ideal donor for a kidney transplantation is a biological sibling.

- Breast cancer is the leading cancer among women.

- The four stages of cervical cancer are stage 0, carcinoma in situ; stage I, cancer confined to the cervix; stage II, cancer extension beyond the cervix but not to pelvic wall; stage III, cancer extension to pelvic wall; stage IV, cancer extension beyond the pelvis or within the bladder or rectum.

- One method of estimating blood loss after a hysterectomy is by counting peripads.

- Transurethral resection of the prostate is the most common procedure for treating benign prostatic hypertrophy.

- In a chest drainage system, the water in the water-seal chamber normally fluctuates with the patient's respirations.

- Placenta previa is the abnormally low implantation of the placenta so that it encroaches on or covers the cervical os.

- Spinal infusion provides spinal stability through a bone graft, usually from the iliac crest, by fusing two or more vertebrae.

- To turn a patient by logrolling, the nurse folds the patient's arms across the chest, extends the patient's legs, places a draw sheet under the patient, and turns the patient by slowly and gently pulling on the draw sheet.

- In complete (total) placenta previa, the placenta covers the cervical os.

- In partial (incomplete or marginal) placenta previa, the placenta covers only a portion of the cervical os.

- A patient who receives any type of transplant must receive an immunosuppressant for life.

- Abruptio placenta is the premature separation of a normally implanted placenta. It may be partial or complete and usually causes abdominal pain and vaginal bleeding.

- Cutis marmorata (mottling or purple skin discoloration) is a transient vasomotor response that occurs primarily in the arms and legs of infants exposed to cold.

- The classic triad of symptoms of preeclampsia are hypertension, edema, and proteinuria. Additional symptoms in severe preeclampsia include hyperreflexia, cerebral and visual disturbances, and epigastric pain.

- The four classifications of mental retardation are mild (educable with an intelligence quotient [IQ] of 50 to 70), moderate (trainable with an IQ of 40 to 50), severe (with an IQ of 20 to 40), and profound (custodial with an IQ under 20).

- In a male patient who has reached puberty, the major complication of mumps is sterility caused by orchitis.

- Pelvic inflammatory disease is a common complication of gonorrhea in women.

- Hirschsprung's disease (congenital megacolon) is the congenital absence of parasympathetic ganglia in the distal portion of the colon and rectum, which results in a lack of peristalsis.

- Ortolani's sign (an audible click or palpable jerk with thigh abduction) confirms congenital hip dislocation in a neonate.

- Scoliosis is the lateral S-shaped curvature of the spine.

- According to Freud, conflicts that arise in the phallic stage (Oedipus or Electra complex) are resolved when the child identifies with the parent of the same sex.

- Signs and symptoms of the secondary stage of syphilis include a rash on the palms and soles, erosion of the oral mucosa, alopecia, and enlarged lymph nodes.

- Alcoholics Anonymous recommends a 12-step program to achieve sobriety.

- The nurse should monitor glucose and electrolyte levels in a patient receiving TPN.

- Signs and symptoms of anorexia nervosa include amenorrhea, excessive weight loss (more than 25% of body weight), lanugo (fine body hair), abdominal distention, and electrolyte disturbances.

- In treating substance abuse, the nurse should realize that the relapse rate is high.

- Alcohol is a CNS depressant.

- A patient who consumes high-tyramine foods while taking an MAO inhibitor may experience a hypertensive crisis, marked by dangerously elevated blood pressure, headache, chills, nausea, and restlessness.

- Serum lithium levels that exceed 1.5 mEq/liter are considered toxic.

- The bell of a stethoscope is used to hear low-pitched sounds, such as heart murmurs.

- A severe complication of a femur fracture is excessive blood loss, resulting in shock.

- To prepare the patient for peritoneal dialysis, the nurse should ask the patient to void, measure the patient's vital signs, place the patient in a supine position, and insert a catheter through the abdominal wall into the peritoneal space.

- If more than 3 liters of dialysate solution return during peritoneal dialysis, the nurse should notify the physician.

- Hemodialysis is the removal of certain elements from the blood by passing heparinized blood through a semipermeable membrane to the dialysate bath, which contains all the important electrolytes in their ideal concentrations.

- *Pneumocystis carinii* pneumonia, a marker disease of AIDS, is caused by a protozoa.

- Gangrene usually affects the digits first and begins with skin color changes that progress from gray-blue to dark brown or black.

- Two types of gangrene exist: dry gangrene, which is uninfected and mummified and tends to self-amputate, and wet gangrene, which is infected, swollen, moist, and painful and spreads more rapidly.

- The diaphragm of the stethoscope is used to hear high-pitched sounds, such as breath sounds.

- A slight blood pressure difference (5 to 10 mm Hg) is normal.

- A weight-bearing transfer is appropriate only for a patient who has at least one strong leg, such as one with hemiplegia or a single leg amputation.

- The nurse should place the blood pressure cuff 1" (2.5 cm) above the antecubital fossa.

- The blood pressure cuff should cover one-third of the patient's upper arm.

- The nurse should use a leg cuff to measure blood pressure in an obese patient.

- If the blood pressure cuff is applied too loosely, the reading will be falsely evelated.

- Ptosis is eyelid drooping.

- Overflow incontinence (voiding of 30 to 60 ml of urine every 15 to 30 minutes) is a sign of bladder distention.

- The first sign of a pressure ulcer is reddened skin that blanches when pressure is applied.

- A tilt table is useful for a patient with a spinal cord injury, orthostatic hypotension, or brain damage because it can move the patient gradually from a horizontal to a vertical (upright) position.

- To perform venipuncture with the least injury to the vessel, the nurse should turn the bevel upward when the vessel's lumen is larger than the needle and turn it downward when the lumen is only slightly larger than the needle.

- To move the patient to the edge of the bed for transfer, follow these steps: (1) Move the patient's head and shoulders toward the edge of bed. (2) Move the patient's feet and legs to the edge of bed (crescent position). (3) Place both arms well under the patient's hip and straighten the back while moving the patient toward the edge of the bed.

- Signs and symptoms of chronic sickle cell anemia include tachycardia, cardiomegaly, systolic and diastolic murmurs, chronic fatigue, hepatomegaly, and splenomegaly.

- Signs and symptoms of sickle cell anemia during early childhood include jaundice, pallor, joint swelling, bone pain, chest pain, ischemic leg ulcers, and an increased susceptibility to infection.

- When being measured for crutches, a patient should wear his or her shoes.

- If a patient misses a menstrual period while taking an oral contraceptive exactly as prescribed, she should continue taking the contraceptive.

- If a patient misses two consecutive menstrual periods while taking an oral contraceptive, she should discontinue the contraceptive and have a pregnancy test.

- If a patient taking an oral contraceptive misses a dose, she should take the pill as soon as she remembers or take two at the next scheduled interval and continue with the normal schedule.

- If a patient taking an oral contraceptive misses two consecutive doses, she should double the dose for 2 days and then resume her normal schedule. Also, she should use an additional birth control method for 1 week.

- A mechanical ventilator, which can maintain ventilation automatically for an extended period, is indicated when a patient cannot maintain a safe oxygen or carbon dioxide level.

- Two types of mechanical ventilators exist: negative-pressure ventilators, which apply negative pressure around the chest wall, and positive-pressure ventilators, which deliver air under pressure to the patient.

- Angina pectoris is characterized by substernal pain that lasts for 2 to 3 minutes. The pain, which is caused by myocardial ischemia, may radiate to the neck, shoulders, or jaw; is described as vise-like or constricting; and may be accompanied by severe apprehension or a feeling of impending doom.

- Anginal pain that persists for more than 20 minutes and is not relieved by nitroglycerin indicates a developing MI.

- The goal of treatment for a patient with angina pectoris is to reduce the heart's workload, thereby reducing the myocardial oxygen demand and preventing MI.

- Nitroglycerin decreases the amount of blood returning to the heart by increasing the capacity of the venous bed, which causes blood to pool in the body.

- The patient should take no more than three nitroglycerin tablets in a 15-minute period.

- Hemodialysis usually is performed 24 hours before kidney transplantation.

- Signs and symptoms of acute kidney transplant rejection are progressive enlargement and tenderness at the transplant site, increased blood pressure, decreased urine output, elevated serum creatinine level, and fever.

- In an infant, one of the first signs of dehydration is sunken fontanelles.

- After a radical mastectomy, the patient's arm should be elevated on a pillow to enhance circulation and prevent edema.

- Postoperative mastectomy care includes teaching the patient arm exercises to facilitate lymph drainage and prevent muscle shortening and shoulder joint contracture.

- Eclampsia is the occurrence of seizures not caused by a cerebral disorder in a patient with preeclampsia.

• A patient who has had a radical mastectomy should help prevent infection by making sure that no blood pressure readings, injections, or venipunctures are performed on the affected arm.

• In placenta previa, bleeding is painless and seldom fatal on the first occasion but becomes heavier with each subsequent episode.

• For a mastectomy patient prone to lymphedema, the hand exercise program can begin shortly after surgery, if pre-scribed. It consists of having the patient open and close her hand tightly six to eight times hourly and perform such tasks as washing her face and combing her hair.

• Treatment for abruptio placentae usually is immediate cesarean section.

• The nurse should transport a hospitalized infant or child in a stroller, wheelchair, or bed, rather than hand-carry the infant or child.

• The nurse should attach a restraint to the bed frame or springs—not to the mattress or side rails.

• Drugs used to treat neonatal withdrawal symptoms include phenobarbital (Luminal), camphorated opium tincture (Paregoric), and diazepam (Valium).

• Signs and symptoms of theophylline toxicity include vomiting, restlessness, and an apical pulse rate over 200 beats/minute.

• The mist in a mist tent should never become so dense that it obscures clear visualization of the patient's respiratory pattern.

• The nurse should teach the parent of a child with croup not to administer cough medication because it may worsen the child's respiratory distress by inhibiting the body's natural response to clear the throat by coughing.

• Infants with Down's syndrome typically display marked hypotonia, floppiness, slanted eyes, excess skin on the back of the neck, flattened bridge of the nose, flat facial features, spade-like hands, short and broad feet, small genitalia, absence of Moro's reflex, and simian crease.

• The nurse should not induce vomiting in a person who has ingested poison and is having seizures or is semiconscious or comatose.

• Public Law 94-247 (Child Abuse and Neglect Act of 1973) requires that suspected cases of child abuse be reported.

• The nurse should suspect sexual abuse in a young patient who has blood in the stool or urine, penile or vaginal discharge, genital trauma that is not readily explained, or a sexually transmitted disease.

• Central venous pressure (CVP), the pressure in the right atrium and the great veins in the thorax, normally ranges from 2 to 8 mm Hg (or 3 to 15 cm of water) and serves as a guide for assessing right-sided cardiac function.

• CVP monitoring is used to assess the need for fluid replacement in seriously ill patients, estimate blood volume deficits, and evaluate circulatory pressure in the right atrium.

• To administer heparin subcutaneously (S.C.), the nurse should follow these steps: (1) Clean—but do not rub—the site with alcohol. (2) Stretch the skin taut or pick up a well-defined skin fold. (3) Hold the shaft of the needle in a dart position. (4) Insert the needle into the skin at a right angle. (5) Firmly depress the plunger, but do not aspirate). (6) Leave the needle in place for 10 seconds. (7) Withdraw the needle gently at the same angle it was inserted. (8) Apply pressure to the injection site with an alcohol pad.

• To prevent deep vein thrombosis after surgery, the nurse should administer 5,000 units of heparin S.C. every 8 to 12 hours, as prescribed.

• Oral anticoagulants, such as warfarin sodium (Coumadin) and dicumarol, disrupt natural blood clotting mechanisms, prevent thrombus formation, and limit the extension of a formed thrombus.

• Anticoagulants cannot dissolve a formed thrombus.

• Anticoagulant therapy is contraindicated in a patient with liver or kidney disease or GI ulcers or one who is not likely to return for follow-up visits.

• The nurse can assess for thrombophlebitis by measuring the patient's affected and unaffected legs and comparing their sizes. The nurse should mark measurement locations with a pen so that the measurements can be taken at the same place each day.

• Drainage of more than 3,000 ml of fluid daily from a nasogastric tube may suggest intestinal obstruction. Yellow drainage with a foul odor may indicate small intestine obstruction.

• For a sigmoidoscopy, the nurse should place the patient in a knee-chest or Sims' position, depending on the physician's preference.

• Preparation for sigmoidoscopy includes administering an enema 1 hour before the examination, warming the scope in warm water or a sterilizer, and draping the patient so that the perineum is exposed.

• Treatment for a patient with bleeding esophageal varices includes administering vasopressin (Pitressin), giving an ice water lavage, aspirating blood from the stomach, using an esophageal tamponade, providing parenteral nutrition, and administering blood transfusions, as needed.

• A trauma victim should not be moved until a patent airway has been established and the cervical spine has been immobilized.

• After a mastectomy, lymphedema may cause a feeling of heaviness in the arm.

• A school-age child faced with dying should be told the truth. The child should receive an explanation of the diagnosis and should be allowed to die in comfort surrounded by family.

• A preschool-age child with a fatal disease is not likely to ask if he or she is going to die but may express anxiety about death through play therapy or other activities. Most developmental theorists recommend helping such a child by responding honestly to questions and providing reassurance that he or she will not be alone.

• It is appropriate for the parents and family to tell their dying child that they will miss him or her and that they are sad because they will be separated.

• An adolescent with a terminal illness should be told the truth about the prognosis, although resentment and denial ("Is it possible that I will live?") are common responses.

• A dying patient should not be given an absolute time left to live but should receive a statement such as "Some people live 3 to 6 months, but others live longer."

• After a child dies, the nurse should give family members time with the body, compliment them (as appropriate) on the excellent care they provided, and give them the name of a person to contact if they have questions.

• Amniocentesis (needle aspiration of amniotic fluid) usually is performed at 15 to 17 weeks' gestation to detect fetal abnormalities.

• For a child over age 1 who has ingested a noncorrosive poison, treatment should include administration of 15 ml of syrup of ipecac mixed in warm water. Tincture of ipecac should not be used because it is stronger than syrup of ipecac and is itself a poison.

- A sign is an objective indication of a disease as perceived by the examining clinician.

- A symptom is a subjective indication of a disease as reported by the patient.

- The amnion is the innermost membrane of the placenta.

- An alcoholic uses alcohol as a way to cope with the stresses of life.

- Theophylline, steroids, and terbutaline commonly are used to treat children with asthma.

- Treatment of a child with celiac disease includes following a lifelong gluten-free diet.

- The ectoderm is the outermost layer of the three primary germ layers of the embryo.

- The human personality operates on three levels: conscious, preconscious, and unconscious.

- Asking an open-ended question is the best way to elicit or clarify information from a patient.

- The failure rate of a contraceptive is determined by the experience of 100 women for 1 year and is expressed as pregnancies per 100 women years.

- The narrowest diameter of the pelvic inlet is the anteroposterior (diagonal conjugate).

- The chorion is the outermost extraembryonic membrane that gives rise to the placenta.

- The corpus luteum secretes large quantities of progesterone.

- From the 8th week of gestation through delivery, the developing cells are termed a *fetus*.

- The diagnosis of autism usually is made when a child reaches age 2.

- In an incomplete abortion, the fetus is expelled but parts of the placenta and membrane remain in the uterus.

- A neonate's head circumference normally is 2 to 3 cm greater than the chest circumference.

- After administering magnesium sulfate to a pregnant patient for hypertension or preterm labor, the nurse should monitor her respiratory rate and deep tendon reflexes.

- During the first hour after birth (the period of reactivity), the neonate is alert and awake.

- When a pregnant patient has undiagnosed vaginal bleeding, vaginal examinations should be avoided until ultrasonography rules out placenta previa.

- After a neonate is delivered, the first nursing action is to establish the neonate's airway.

- Nursing interventions for a patient with placenta previa include positioning the patient on her left side for maximum fetal perfusion, monitoring fetal heart tones, and administering I.V. fluids and oxygen, as needed.

- When taking a child's temperature rectally, the nurse should insert the thermometer only ½" (1.3 cm).

- The specific gravity of a neonate's urine is 1.003 to 1.030. A lower specific gravity suggests overhydration; a higher one suggests dehydration.

- During the oral stage of development (from age 1 to 18 months), the infant receives satisfaction, relieves tension, and derives pleasure from sucking and chewing.

- Defense mechanisms serve as protectors of the personality by reducing stress and anxiety.

• A Milwaukee brace, which is used for patients with structural scoliosis, helps halt the progression of spinal curvature by providing longitudinal traction and lateral pressure. It should be worn 23 hours a day.

• Suppression is the voluntary act of excluding anxiety- or stress-producing thoughts from the conscious.

• Most infants are weighed and measured monthly for the first 6 months of life.

• The neonatal period extends from birth to day 28. It may also be called the first 4 weeks or first month of life.

• The infancy period lasts from birth to age 1.

• The toddler stage encompasses ages 1 to 3 years.

• Children with chronic protein-calorie malnutrition are small for their age, physically inactive, mentally sluggish, and susceptible to infections.

• Before breast-feeding, the mother should clean each nipple with a cotton ball soaked in sterile water, starting at the nipple and cleaning outward in a circular motion.

• Breast-feeding should begin as soon as possible after delivery. The neonate should be allowed to feed for 10 to 15 minutes on each breast.

• A patient who is breast-feeding should rub a mild emollient cream or a few drops of breast milk (or colostrum) on the nipples to prevent them from cracking.

• Breast-feeding mothers should increase their fluid intake to 2.5 to 3 qt (2,500 to 3,000 ml) daily.

• Psychodrama is a therapeutic technique used with groups to help participants gain new perception and self-awareness by acting out their own or assigned problems.

- Maslow's hierarchy of needs must be met in the following order: physiologic (oxygen, food, water, sex, rest, and comfort), safety and security, love and belonging, self-esteem and recognition, and self-actualization.

- A patient who is taking disulfiram (Antabuse) must avoid ingesting products that contain alcohol, such as cough syrup and sauces and soups made with cooking wine.

- A patient who is admitted involuntarily to a psychiatric hospital loses the right to sign out against medical advice.

- "People who live in glass houses should not throw stones" and "A rolling stone gathers no moss" are examples of proverbs.

- Proverbs are used in a psychiatric interview to determine a patient's ability for abstract thinking. (Schizophrenic patients think in concrete terms and might interpret the glass house proverb as "If you throw a stone in a glass house, the house will break.")

- Signs of lithium toxicity are diarrhea, tremors, nausea, muscle weakness, ataxia, and confusion.

- A labile affect is characterized by rapid shifts of emotions and mood.

- Amnesia is a loss of memory from an organic or inorganic cause.

- A person with borderline personality disorder is demanding and judgmental in interpersonal relationships.

- Disulfiram (Antabuse) should not be taken concurrently with metronidazole (Flagyl) because they may interact, causing a psychotic reaction.

- Congenital hip dysplasia is the most common disorder of the hip joint in a patient under age 3.

• Histrionic personality disorder is defined as excessive attention-seeking and emotional behavior by people who are seeking praise and approval from others.

• To relieve postoperative hiccups, the patient should rebreathe into a paper bag.

• Apgar scoring is used to assess a neonate's vital functioning.

• Apgar scoring is done at 1 and 5 minutes after birth.

• After feeding an infant with a cleft lip or palate, the nurse should rinse the infant's mouth with sterile water.

• An infant with a cleft palate is at increased risk of developing otitis media.

• When examining an infant's ear with an otoscope, the nurse should pull the earlobe down and back.

• The nurse should place oral medication to the side of the mouth in an infant who has had corrective surgery for a cleft lip or palate.

• The nurse should position a child with meningococcal meningitis on the side if opisthotonos (back arching) occurs.

• Between ages 2 and 3 years, a child engages in parallel play and begins to interact with others.

• For a child with ascites from a chronic liver disease, the nurse should use semi-Fowler's position to promote respiratory functioning.

• An autistic child is difficult to understand because of withdrawal, unresponsiveness, and severely impaired speech.

• In a toddler, the first signs of respiratory distress are increased respiratory and pulse rates.

- Toilet training usually is unsuccessful before ages 15 to 18 months because sphincter control develops at this age.

- The nurse instills silver nitrate or erythromycin in the neonate's eyes primarily to prevent blindness caused by gonorrhea.

- Because gonorrhea is asymptomatic and progresses without detection in most teenage girls, their fallopian tubes can be damaged.

- During the initial interview and treatment of a patient with syphilis, the patient's sexual contacts should be identified.

- The nurse should not administer morphine to a patient whose respiratory rate has fallen below 12 breaths per minute.

- The nurse should administer oxygen to a patient only if it has been prescribed by a physician.

- Flavoxate hydrochloride (Urispas) is classified as a urinary tract spasmolytic.

- Hypotension is a sign of cardiogenic shock in a patient with an MI.

- In hypovolemic shock, the pulse rate increases and the blood pressure decreases.

- For a patient with an MI, the nurse should monitor fluid intake and output meticulously because too little intake causes dehydration and too much may cause pulmonary edema.

- Nitroglycerin relaxes smooth muscle, causing vasodilation and relieving the chest pain associated with MI and angina.

- The diagnosis of an acute MI is based on the patient's signs and symptoms, ECG tracings, and serum enzyme studies.

• Arrhythmias are the predominant problem during the first 48 hours after an MI.

• The nurse should irrigate a gastric tube with normal saline solution.

• When caring for a patient with a nasogastric tube, the nurse should apply a water-soluble lubricant to the nostril to prevent soreness.

• Asparaginase, an enzyme that inhibits deoxyribonucleic acid (DNA) and protein synthesis, is used to treat acute lymphocytic leukemia.

• To relieve a patient's sore throat caused by gastric tube irritation, the nurse should provide anesthetic lozenges, as prescribed.

• For the first 12 to 24 hours after gastric surgery, stomach contents (obtained by suctioning) are brown.

• During gastric lavage, a nasogastric tube is inserted, the stomach is flushed, and ingested substances are removed through the tube.

• After gastric suctioning is discontinued, a patient recovering from a subtotal gastrectomy should receive a clear fluid diet.

• In documenting drainage on a surgical dressing, the nurse should include the size, color, and consistency of the drainage—for example, "10 mm of brown mucoid drainage noted on dressing."

• Stress in the work environment has been linked to the development of peptic ulcers.

• The classic signs and symptoms of pyloric stenosis are a palpable olive-sized mass in the right upper quadrant, strong peristaltic movements from left to right during meals, and projectile vomiting.

- The preferred site for a permanent colostomy is the descending colon.

- Although rare, electroconvulsive therapy (ECT) can cause arrhythmias and death.

- A patient who is scheduled for ECT should receive nothing by mouth after midnight to prevent aspiration while under anesthesia.

- Valvular insufficiency in the veins commonly causes varicosity.

- A patient with a colostomy should restrict fat and fibrous foods and should avoid foods that can obstruct the stoma, such as corn, nuts, and cabbage.

- A patient receiving chemotherapy is placed on reverse isolation because the WBC count may be depressed.

- Symptoms of mitral valve stenosis are caused by improper emptying of the left atrium.

- Persistent bleeding after open heart surgery may require protamine sulfate administration to reverse the effects of heparin sodium (Liquaemin) used during surgery.

- The nurse should teach a patient with congestive heart failure (CHF) to take digitalis and other drugs as prescribed, restrict sodium intake, restrict fluids as prescribed, get adequate rest, gradually increase walking and other activities, avoid temperature extremes, report signs of CHF recurrence, and keep regular physician appointments.

- The nurse should check and maintain the patency of all connections for a chest tube. If an air leak is detected, the nurse should add water to the suction system.

- In two-person cardiopulmonary resuscitation (CPR), the rescuers should administer 60 chest compressions per minute and 1 breath for every 5 compressions.

- Mitral valve stenosis can result from rheumatic fever.

- Atelectasis is incomplete expansion of lung segments or lobules (clusters of alveoli), which may result in lung collapse.

- The nurse should instruct a patient with an ileal conduit to empty the collection device frequently because the weight of the urine may cause the device to slip from the skin.

- A patient who is receiving CPR should be placed on a solid, flat surface.

- Brain damage occurs in 4 to 6 minutes after cardiopulmonary function ceases.

- Climacteric is the transition period during which a woman's reproductive function diminishes and gradually disappears.

- Menses is the normal flow of blood and decidua that occurs during menstruation.

- To elicit Babinski's reflex, the nurse strokes the sole of the patient's foot with a moderately sharp object, such as a thumbnail.

- In a positive Babinski's reflex, the great toe dorsiflexes and the other toes fan out.

- Milk is contraindicated for a patient with an ulcer because its high calcium content stimulates gastric acid secretion.

- When assessing a patient for bladder distention, the nurse should check the contour of the lower abdomen for a rounded mass above the symphysis pubis.

- A patient who tests positive for HIV has been exposed to the virus associated with AIDS but does not necessarily have AIDS.

- A common complication after a prostatectomy is circulatory failure caused by bleeding.

- Most neonates born with HIV-positive blood develop AIDS within 2 to 4 months.

- Because the HIV virus has been cultured in breast milk, it could be transmitted by an HIV-positive mother who breast-feeds her infant.

- In right-sided heart failure, a major focus of nursing care is decreasing the heart's work load.

- Signs and symptoms of digitalis toxicity include vomiting, confusion, and arrhythmias.

- The best way to prevent pressure ulcers is to reposition the bedridden patient every 2 hours.

- An asthma attack typically begins with wheezing, coughing, and increasing respiratory distress.

- In a patient recovering from a tonsillectomy, frequent swallowing suggests hemorrhage.

- Ileostomies and Hartman colostomies are permanent stomas. Loop colostomies and double-barrel colostomies are temporary ones.

- A patient with an ileostomy should eat foods such as spinach and parsley because they act as intestinal tract deodorizers.

- An adrenalectomy can decrease steroid production, which can cause extensive sodium and water loss.

- A fever in the first 24 hours postpartum may be caused by dehydration, rather than infection.

- Antiembolism stockings decompress the superficial blood vessels, thereby preventing thrombus formation.

- Before administering morphine sulfate (Duramorph) to a patient suspected of having an MI, the nurse should check the patient's respiratory rate. If it is not greater than 12 breaths per minute, the nurse should keep emergency equipment readily available for intubation if respiratory depression occurs.

- In a healthy person, the amount of fluid taken in should roughly equal the amount lost.

- Preterm infants or infants who cannot maintain a skin temperature of at least 97.6° F (36.4° C) should receive care in an incubator (Isolette) or a radiant warmer. In a radiant warmer, a heat-sensitive probe taped to the infant's skin activates the heater unit automatically to maintain the desired temperature.

- After a patient undergoes femoral-popliteal bypass graft, the nurse must closely monitor peripheral pulses and circulation.

- After a femoral-popliteal bypass graft, a patient initially should maintain a semi-Fowler's position to avoid flexion of the graft site. Before discharge, the nurse should instruct the patient to avoid the positions that put pressure on the graft site until the next follow-up visit.

- Of the five senses, hearing is the last to be lost in a patient who is entering a coma.

- The most convenient veins for venipuncture in an adult patient are the basilic and median cubital veins in the antecubital space.

- Cholelithiasis produces an enlarged, edematous gallbladder with multiple stones, and an elevated bilirubin level.

- The antiviral agent azidothymidine (Retrovir) has been successful in slowing HIV replication, thereby slowing the development of AIDS.

- Severe rheumatoid arthritis produces marked edema and congestion, which cause spindle-shaped joints and severe flexion deformities.

- A patient with AIDS should observe sexual precautions, such as abstinence or condom use.

- If a radioactive implant becomes dislodged, the nurse should retrieve it with tongs, place it in a lead-shielded container, and notify the radiology department.

- A patient undergoing radiation therapy should pat the skin dry to avoid abrasions that could easily become infected in such an immunocompromised patient.

- During radiation therapy, a patient should have frequent blood tests, especially WBC and platelet counts.

- The nurse should administer an aluminum hydroxide antacid at least 1 hour after an enteric-coated medication because it can cause premature release of the enteric-coated medication in the stomach.

- By age 1 year, an infant has tripled its birth weight, can sit alone and roll over, and has eight teeth.

- Acid-base balance refers to the body's hydrogen ion concentration, a measure of the ratio of carbonic acid to bicarbonate (1 part carbonic acid to 20 parts bicarbonate).

- Buffers are substances in the blood that have acidic and basic properties.

- Metabolic acidosis results from an abnormal loss of bicarbonate or excessive production or retention of acid ions.

- Hemianopia is defective vision or blindness in half the visual field of one or both eyes.

- Two common manifestations of SLE are early-morning joint stiffness and facial erythema in a butterfly pattern.

- After a total knee replacement, the patient should remain in the semi-Fowler's position with the affected leg elevated.

- When caring for a patient receiving transpyloric feedings, the nurse should monitor for dumping syndrome and hypovolemic shock because the stomach is being bypassed.

- From 2 to 3 hours before beginning a tube feeding, the nurse should aspirate the patient's stomach contents to verify adequate gastric emptying.

- If a TPN infusion must be interrupted, the nurse should administer dextrose 5% in water (D_5W) at a similar rate because abrupt cessation can result in hypoglycemia.

- People with type O blood are known as universal donors.

- People with type AB blood are known as universal recipients.

- In setting-sun sign, which reflects increased intracranial pressure in children, the eyes are forced downward so that a rim of sclera shows above the irises.

- Phenytoin (Dilantin) is the drug of choice in treating status epilepticus.

- Disequilibrium syndrome, manifested by nausea, vomiting, restlessness, and twitching, occurs in patients undergoing dialysis and results from a rapid fluid shift.

- ECT therapy usually is used for patients with severe depression that does not respond to drug therapy.

- For ECT to be effective, the patient should receive 6 to 12 treatments at a rate of two or three per week.

- An indication that spinal shock is resolving is the return of reflex activity in the legs and arms below the level of the injury.

• Hypovolemia is the most common and fatal complication of severe acute pancreatitis.

• Oral care for a patient with stomatitis includes mouth rinses with a mixture of equal parts of hydrogen peroxide and water three times daily.

• Hertz (Hz) is the unit of measure of sound frequency.

• In otitis media, the tympanic membrane is bright red and lacks a light reflex (cone of light).

• Hearing protection is required when the sound intensity exceeds 84 dB; double hearing protection is required if it exceeds 104 dB.

• In pericardiocentesis, fluid is aspirated from the pericardial sac for analysis or relief of cardiac tamponade.

• During labor, the resting phase between contractions should be at least 30 seconds.

• Urticaria is an early sign of hemolytic transfusion reaction.

• During peritoneal dialysis, a return of brown dialysate suggests bowel perforation and requires immediate physician notification.

• An early sign of ketoacidosis is polyuria, which results from osmotic diuresis.

• Infants with hydrocephalus usually have a high-pitched, shrill cry.

• Vitamin K (Synkayvite) is used to treat warfarin (Coumadin) overdose.

• Prothrombin, a clotting factor, is produced in the liver.

• Aspirated red bone marrow usually appears rust-red with visible fatty material and white bone fragments.

- If a patient is menstruating when a urine sample is collected, the nurse should note this on the laboratory slip.

- During lumbar puncture, the nurse must note the initial intracranial pressure and the cerebrospinal fluid color.

- A patient who cannot cough to provide a sputum sample for culture may require a heated aerosol treatment.

- The Dick test detects scarlet fever antigens and immunity or susceptibility to scarlet fever. A positive result indicates no immunity; a negative result indicates immunity.

- The Schick test detects diphtheria antigens and immunity or susceptibility to diphtheria. A positive result indicates no immunity; a negative result indicates immunity.

- The recommended adult dosage of sucralfate (Carafate) for duodenal ulcer is 1 g (one tablet) four times a day 1 hour before meals and at bedtime.

- If eye ointment and eye drops must be instilled in the same eye, the eye drops should be instilled first.

- When leaving an isolation room, the nurse should remove the gloves before the mask because fewer pathogens are on the mask.

- Lochia rubra is the vaginal discharge of almost pure blood that occurs during the first few days after childbirth.

- Lochia serosa is the serous vaginal discharge that occurs about 4 or 5 days after childbirth.

- Lochia alba is the vaginal discharge of decreased blood and increased leukocytes that is the final stage of lochia after childbirth.

- A patient with facial burns or smoke or heat inhalation should be admitted to the hospital for 24 hours for observation for delayed tracheal edema.

• Patient preparation for a colostomy includes nothing by mouth overnight, bowel preparation, and a cleansing enema.

• Skeletal traction is applied to a bone using wire pins or tongs. It is the most effective means of traction.

• Two stages of physiologic changes take place with burn injuries: the hypovolemic stage, during which intravascular fluid shifts into the interstitial space, and the diuretic stage, during which capillary integrity and intravascular volume are restored, usually 48 to 72 hours after the injury.

• The nurse should change TPN tubing every 24 hours and the injection site every 3 days.

• The TPN solution should be stored in a refrigerator and removed 30 to 60 minutes before use because delivery of a chilled solution can cause pain, hypothermia, venous spasm, and venous constriction.

• Colostrum (the precursor of milk) is the first secretion from a maternity patient's breasts.

• The length of the uterus increases from 2.6" (6.5 cm) before pregnancy to 12.8" (32 cm) at term.

• Because the true conjugate (the smallest inlet measurement of the pelvis) cannot be measured directly, the diagonal conjugate, which can be measured directly, is used to estimate the true conjugate.

• The smallest outlet measurement of the pelvis is the intertuberous diameter, which is the transverse diameter between the ischial tuberosities.

• Electronic fetal monitoring is used to assess fetal well-being during labor. If compromised fetal status is suspected, fetal blood pH may be evaluated by obtaining a scalp sample.

• A patient whose carbon monoxide level falls between 20% and 30% should be treated with 100% humidified oxygen.

- When in the room of a patient in isolation for tuberculosis, staff members and visitors should wear an ultrafilter mask.

- When providing skin care at the pin insertion site, the nurse's primary concern is prevention of osteomyelitis. Prevention of skin breakdown is a secondary concern.

- A diagnosis of cystic fibrosis is confirmed by a sweat test. Sodium and chloride concentrations of 50 to 60 mEq/L strongly suggest cystic fibrosis.

- In a patient who has had an amputation, moist skin may signify venous stasis; dry skin may indicate arterial obstruction.

- Medication is not routinely injected I.M. into edematous tissue because it may not be absorbed.

- In a patient receiving dialysis, an internal shunt is working if the nurse can feel a thrill on palpation or hear a bruit on auscultation.

- In a patient with viral hepatitis, the parenchymal or Kupffer's cells of the liver become severely inflamed, enlarged, and necrotic.

- Early signs of AIDS include fatigue, night sweats, enlarged lymph nodes, anorexia, weight loss, pallor, and fever.

- When caring for a patient with a radioactive implant, health care workers should stay as far away from the radiation source as possible and should remember the axiom "If you double the distance, you quarter the dose."

- During the manic phase of a bipolar affective disorder, nursing care is directed at slowing the patient because death may result from self-induced exhaustion or injury.

- The nursing care plan for a patient with Alzheimer's disease should focus on safety measures.

- Growth disturbances, such as bone shortening or overgrowth, may occur in children as a result of a fracture of the epiphyseal plate.

- In an emergency delivery, enough pressure should be applied to the emerging fetus's head to guide the descent and prevent a rapid change in pressure within the molded fetal skull.

- A multiparous woman is prone to bleeding after delivery because her uterine muscles may be overstretched and may not contract efficiently.

- Normal values for BUN range from 10 to 20 mg/dl.

- The cardinal signs of Parkinson's disease are muscle rigidity, a tremor that begins in the fingers, and akinesia.

- In a patient with Parkinson's disease, levodopa (Dopar) is prescribed to compensate for the dopamine deficiency.

- A patient with multiple sclerosis is at increased risk of developing pressure ulcers.

- Pill-rolling tremor is a classic sign of Parkinson's disease.

- For a patient with Parkinson's disease, nursing interventions are palliative.

- Fat embolism, a serious complication of a long bone fracture, produces fever, tachycardia, tachypnea, and anxiety.

- Metrorrhagia (bleeding between menstrual periods) may be the first sign of cervical cancer.

- In a rape case, the patient is the primary concern followed by the medicolegal considerations.

- A patient taking phenytoin sodium (Dilantin) must practice good dental hygiene because of the risk of developing gingival hyperplasia.

- When caring for a comatose patient, the nurse should explain each action to the patient in a normal voice.

- When cleaning dentures, the sink should be lined with a washcloth.

- A patient should void within 8 hours after surgery.

- An EEG identifies normal and abnormal brain waves.

- The classic sign of a petit mal seizure is a vacant facial expression.

- Migraine headaches are manifested as persistent, severe pain usually in the temporal region.

- A patient in a bladder retraining program should void every 2 hours during the day and twice at night.

- A decrease in level of consciousness is a cardinal sign of increased intracranial pressure.

- Stool samples for ova and parasite tests should be delivered to the laboratory without delay or refrigeration.

- The autonomic nervous system regulates the cardiovascular and respiratory systems.

- Ergotamine tartrate (Ergomar) is most effective when taken during the prodromal phase of a migraine or vascular headache.

- Treatment of acute pancreatitis includes nasogastric suctioning and meperidine (Demerol) for pain.

- Symptoms of hiatal hernia include a feeling of fullness in the upper abdomen or chest, heartburn, and pain similar to that of angina pectoralis.

- The incidence of cholelithiasis is higher in women who have had children than in any other group.

- An acetaminophen (Tylenol) overdose can severely damage the liver.

- The prominent clinical signs of advanced cirrhosis are ascites and jaundice.

- The first symptom of pancreatitis is steady epigastric pain that radiates from the umbilical area.

- *Somnambulism* is the medical term for sleepwalking.

- Epinephrine (Adrenalin) is a vasoconstrictor.

- An untreated liver laceration or rupture can rapidly progress to hypovolemic shock.

- Obstipation is extreme, intractable constipation caused by an intestinal obstruction.

- When providing tracheostomy care, the nurse should insert the catheter gently into the tracheostomy tube. When withdrawing the catheter, the nurse should apply intermittent suction for no more than 15 seconds and use a slight twisting motion.

- A low-residue diet includes such foods as roasted chicken, rice, and pasta.

- A rectal tube's balloon should be deflated for 20 to 30 minutes every 8 hours.

- Definitive tests for diagnosing cancer are biopsy and cytologic examination of the specimen.

- Patients in a maintenance program for narcotic abstinence syndrome receive 2.5 to 10 mg of methadone hydrochloride (Dolophine) dissolved in 120 ml of orange juice or reconstituted powdered citrus drink every 6 to 8 hours.

- Arthrography requires injection of a contrast medium and can identify joint abnormalities.

- Brompton's cocktail is prescribed for patients with terminal cancer to help relieve pain.

- A patient's bed bath should proceed in this order: face, neck, arms, hands, chest, abdomen, back, legs, perineum.

- When lifting and moving a patient, the nurse should use the upper leg muscles most to prevent injury.

- A sarcoma is a malignant tumor in connective tissue.

- Aluminum hydroxide (Amphojel) neutralizes gastric acid.

- Subluxation is a partial dislocation or a separation and spontaneous reduction of a joint.

- Patient preparation for cholecystography includes ingestion of a contrast medium and a low-fat evening meal.

- Barbiturates can cause confusion and delirium in an elderly patient with organic brain disorder.

- In a patient with arthritis, physical therapy is indicated to promote optimal functioning.

- Most patients with type A hepatitis are anicteric (without jaundice) and lack symptoms, but some develop headaches, anorexia, fatigue, fever, and respiratory tract infection.

- During occupied bed changes, the patient should be covered with a bath blanket to promote warmth and prevent exposure.

- In the preicteric phase, hepatitis A is highly contagious.

- Enteric precautions are required for a patient with hepatitis A.

- Cholecystography is ineffective in a patient with jaundice caused by a gallbladder disease because the liver cells cannot transport the contrast medium to the biliary tract.

- Anticipatory grief is mourning that occurs for an extended time when one realizes that death is inevitable.

- Dehydration is a concern in a patient with diabetes insipidus because this disorder causes polyuria.

- A reducible hernia is one in which the protruding mass can be placed back into the abdomen.

- The following foods can alter stool color: beets (red), cocoa (dark red or brown), licorice (black), spinach (green), and meat protein (dark brown).

- Stress management is a short-range goal of psychotherapy.

- The mood most frequently experienced by a patient with organic brain syndrome is irritability.

- Creative intuition is controlled by the right side of the brain.

- Methohexital sodium (Brevital Sodium) is the general anesthetic administered to patient scheduled for ECT.

- Airway maintenance is the priority nursing intervention during ECT.

- The decision to use restraints should be based on the patient's safety needs.

- Diphenhydramine hydrochloride (Benadryl) relieves the extrapyramidal adverse effects of psychotropic medications.

- A patient who is stabilized on lithium (Eskalith) should have blood lithium levels measured every 1½ to 2 months.

- To prevent purple glove syndrome, the nurse should not administer I.V. phenytoin (Dilantin) through a vein in the back of the hand but should select a larger vessel.

- A placebo stimulates endorphins, which in turn raise the pain threshold in the brain.

- The primary purpose of psychotropic medications is to decrease the patient's symptoms sufficiently to allow participation in therapy.

- Manipulation is considered a maladaptive method of meeting one's needs because it disregards the needs and feelings of others.

- A patient who develops symptoms of lithium toxicity should discontinue the medication and call the physician.

- A patient taking lithium (Eskalith) for bipolar affective disorder must maintain a balanced diet with adequate salt intake.

- A patient who constantly seeks approval from staff members and other patients is demonstrating dependent behavior.

- During stage III of anesthesia (surgical anesthesia), unconsciousness occurs and surgery is permitted.

- Alcoholics Anonymous advocates total abstinence.

- Methylphenidate hydrochloride (Ritalin) is the drug of choice for treating attention deficit disorder in hyperactive children.

- Setting limits is the most effective way to control manipulative behavior.

- Violent outbursts are common in a patient with borderline personality disorder.

- When working with a depressed patient, the nurse should explore meaningful losses.

- An illusion is a sensory experience that is misinterpreted but based on fact.

- Anxiety is nonspecific; fear is specific.

- Extrapyramidal adverse effects are common in patients taking psychotropic medications.

- The nurse should encourage an angry patient to develop a physical exercise program as a way to ventilate feelings.

- Depression can be abnormal if it is characterized by exaggerated feelings of sadness, melancholy, dejection, worthlessness, and hopelessness that are inappropriate or out of proportion to reality.

- Free-floating anxiety is anxiousness with generalized apprehension and pessimism for unknown reasons.

- In a patient experiencing intense anxiety, the fight-or-flight reaction (alarm reflex) may take over.

- The fight-or-flight reaction is a sympathetic nervous system response.

- Confabulation is the use of imaginary experiences or made-up information to fill missing gaps of memory.

- When starting a therapeutic relationship with a patient, the nurse should explain that the purpose of the therapy is to produce a positive change.

- A basic assumption of psychoanalytic theory is that all behavior has meaning.

- TPN solutions contain high levels of glucose, amino acids, and electrolytes.

- Types of regional anesthesia include spinal, caudal, intercostal, epidural, and brachial plexus.

- Masturbation in prepubescent children and adolescents is considered a normal activity at these developmental stages.

- The first step in managing a drug overdose or drug toxicity is to establish and maintain an airway.

- Catharsis is the expression of deep feelings and emotions.

- Respiratory paralysis occurs in stage IV of anesthesia (toxic stage).

- Neonates delivered by cesarean section have a higher incidence of respiratory distress syndrome.

- The nurse should suggest ambulation to a postpartal patient who complains of gas pain and flatulence.

- Massaging the uterus helps stimulate contractions after the placenta is delivered.

- When providing phototherapy to an infant, the nurse should cover the infant's eyes and genital area.

- In stage I of anesthesia, consciousness is maintained and is characterized by tranquility.

- Dyspnea and sharp, stabbing pain that increases with respiration are symptoms of pleurisy, which can be a complication of pneumonia or TB.

- Bronchovesicular breath sounds in peripheral lung fields are abnormal and suggest pneumonia.

- Wheezing is an abnormal, high-pitched breath sound that is accentuated on expiration.

- Wax or a foreign body in the ear should be gently flushed out by irrigation with warm saline solution.

- For a patient whose hearing aid is "not working," the nurse should check the switch first to see if it is turned on and then should check the batteries.

- The nurse should grade hyperactive biceps and triceps reflexes as +4.

- Vertigo is the major symptom of a patient with an inner ear infection or disease.

✓• Loud talking is a sign of hearing impairment.

• A patient with an upper respiratory tract infection should blow the nose with both nostrils open.

• Classic symptoms of glaucoma are halos around lights, headache, and chronic eye pain.

• Dentin is the chief substance (or tissue) that surrounds the teeth.

• An infant with gastroesophageal reflux should receive formula thickened with cereal.

• A patient who has had a cataract removed can begin most normal activities in 3 or 4 days; however, the patient should not bend and lift until a physician approves these activities.

• If two eye medications are prescribed for twice-daily instillation, they should be administered 5 minutes apart.

• Symptoms of corneal transplant rejection include eye irritation and decreasing visual field.

• A child should have a fluoride treatment twice a year.

• Wisdom teeth appear between ages 17 and 21.

• The narcotic antagonist naloxone (Narcan) may be given to a neonate to correct respiratory depression caused by narcotic administration to the mother during labor.

• Symptoms of respiratory distress syndrome in a neonate include expiratory grunting or whining, sandpaper breath sounds, and seesaw retractions.

• In a postoperative patient, forcing fluids helps prevent constipation.

• Cerebral palsy presents as asymmetrical movement, irritability, and excessive feeble crying in a long, thin infant.

- According to the pleasure principle, the psyche seeks pleasure and avoids unpleasant experiences, regardless of the consequences.

- The nurse should assess a breech-birth neonate for hydrocephalus, hematomas, fractures, and other anomalies caused by birth trauma.

- Children ages 3 to 5 years do not conceive of death in final terms but do fear separation from parents.

- Children ages 5 to 9 years view death as a destructive force or, conversely, as an angel coming in the night. They accept death as a final state but do not believe that they are targets.

- A conversion disorder allows a patient to resolve a psychological conflict through the loss of a specific physical function—for example, by paralysis, blindness, or inability to swallow. This loss of function is involuntary, but diagnostic tests show no organic cause.

- Grave's disease (hyperthyroidism) is manifested by weight loss, nervousness, dyspnea, palpitations, heat intolerance, increased thirst, exophthalmos, and goiter.

- When a patient is admitted to the unit in active labor, the nurse's first steps should be to take her vital signs and listen for fetal heart tones.

- In a neonate, long, brittle fingernails are a sign of postmaturity.

- Desquamation (skin peeling) is common in postmature neonates.

- The four types of lipoprotein are chylomicrons (the lowest-density lipoproteins), very low-density liproproteins (VLDLs), low-density lipoproteins (LDLs), and high-density lipoproteins (HDLs). Health care professionals use cholesterol level fractionization to assess a patient's risk of coronary artery disease.

- Greenstick fractures are the most common fractures in children.

- The nurse must administer care in accordance with standards of care established by the American Nursing Association, state regulations, and facility policy.

- The kilocalorie (kcal) is a unit of energy measurement that represents the amount of heat needed to raise the temperature of 1 kg of water 1º C.

- A child with measles requires respiratory isolation.

- As nutrients move through the body, they undergo ingestion, digestion, absorption, transport, cell metabolism, and excretion.

- The body metabolizes alcohol at a fixed rate regardless of serum concentration.

- In an alcoholic beverage, its proof reflects its percentage of alcohol multiplied by 2. For example, a 100-proof beverage contains 50% alcohol.

- If a patient taking amphotericin B (Fungizone) bladder irrigations for a fungal infection develops systemic candidiasis and must receive I.V. fluconazole (Diflucan), the irrigations can be discontinued because fluconazole covers the bladder infection as well.

- Patients with adult respiratory distress syndrome can have high peak inspiratory pressures. Therefore, the nurse should monitor them closely for signs of spontaneous pneumothorax, such as acute deterioration in oxygenation, absence of breath sounds on the affected side, and subcutaneous air beginning on the affected side.

- Adverse reactions to cyclosporine (Sandimmune) include renal and hepatic toxicity, CNS changes (confusion and delirium), GI bleeding, and hypertension.

- Osteoporosis is a metabolic bone disorder in which the rate of bone resorption exceeds the rate of bone formation.

- The hallmark of ulcerative colitis is recurrent bloody diarrhea, which commonly contains pus and mucus, that alternates with asymptomatic remissions.

- Safe sexual practices include massaging, hugging, body rubbing, friendly kissing (dry), masturbating, hand-to-genital touching, wearing a condom, and limiting the numbers of sexual partners.

- Immunosuppressed patients who contract cytomegalovirus (CMV) are at risk for CMV pneumonia and septicemia, which can be fatal.

- A living will is a witnessed document that states a patient's desire for certain types of care and treatment, which depends on that patient's wishes and views on quality of life.

- The nurse should flush a peripheral heparin lock every 8 hours and as needed with normal saline solution to maintain patency.

- Urinary tract infections (UTIs) can produce urinary urgency and frequency, dysuria, abdominal cramps or bladder spasms, and urethral itching.

- A mother should allow her infant to breast-feed until he or she is satisfied. This time may vary from 5 to 20 minutes.

- Mammography is a radiographic technique used to detect breast cysts or tumors, especially those not palpable on physical examination.

- To promote early detection of testicular cancer, palpate the testes during routine physical examinations and encourage the patient to perform monthly self-examinations.

- Quality assurance is a method of determining whether nursing actions and practices meets established standards.

- The five rights of medication administration are the right patient, right medication, right dose, right route of administration, and right time.

- The purpose of the evaluation phase of the nursing process is to determine whether nursing interventions have enabled the patient to meet desired goals.

- Outside of the hospital setting, only the sublingual and translingual forms of nitroglycerin should be used to relieve acute anginal attacks.

- The implementation phase of the nursing process involves recording the patient's response to the nursing plan, putting the nursing plan into action, delegating specific nursing interventions, and coordinating the patient's activities.

- The Patient's Bill of Rights offers guidance and protection to patients by stating the responsibilities of the hospital and its staff toward patients and their families during hospitalization.

- To minimize the omission and distortion of facts, the nurse should record information as soon as it is gathered.

- When assessing a patient's health history, the nurse should record the current illness chronologically, beginning with the onset of the problem and continuing to the present.

- Components of the problem-oriented record are the initial data base, problem list, and progress note.

- Chlordiazepoxide hydrochloride (Librium) is the drug of choice for treating alcohol withdrawal symptoms.

- For a patient at risk of alcohol withdrawal, the nurse should assess the pulse rate and blood pressure every 2 hours for the first 12 hours, every 4 hours for the next 24 hours, and every 6 hours thereafter (unless the patient's condition becomes unstable).

• Alcohol detoxification is most successful when carried out in a structured environment by a supportive, nonjudgmental staff.

• A high level of hepatitis B serum marker (HBsAg) for 3 months or more after the onset of acute hepatitis B infection suggests the development of chronic hepatitis or a carrier status.

• Neurogenic bladder dysfunction results from disruption of nerve transmission to the bladder and may be caused by some spinal cord injuries, diabetes, or multiple sclerosis.

• The nurse should follow these guidelines when caring for a patient who is experiencing alcohol withdrawal: Maintain a calm environment, keep intrusions to a minimum, speak slowly and calmly, adjust lighting to prevent shadows and glare, call the patient by name, and have a friend or family member stay with the patient if possible.

• The therapeutic regimen for an alcoholic patient includes folic acid, thiamine, and multivitamin supplements as well as adequate food and fluids.

• A patient addicted to opiates (drugs derived from poppy seeds, such as heroin and morphine) typically experiences withdrawal symptoms within 12 hours after the last dose. The severest symptoms occur within 48 hours and decrease over the next 2 weeks.

• Oxygen and carbon dioxide move between the lungs and the bloodstream by diffusion.

• To grade the severity of dyspnea, the nurse may use this system: grade 1, shortness of breath with mild exertion, such as walking up steps; grade 2, shortness of breath when walking a short distance at a normal pace on level ground; grade 3, shortness of breath with mild daily activity, such as shaving; grade 4, shortness of breath when supine (orthopnea).

• A patient with Crohn's disease should consume a diet low in residue, fiber, and fat and high in calories, proteins, and carbohydrates and should take vitamin supplements (especially vitamin K).

• A Logan bar is used postoperatively to prevent suture line strain in a child who has had a cleft lip repair.

• In the three-bottle urine collection method, the patient cleans the meatus and urinates 10 to 15 ml in the first bottle and 15 to 30 ml (midstream) in the second bottle. Then the physician performs prostatic massage, and the patient voids into the third bottle.

• Findings in the three-bottle urine collection method are interpreted as follows: pus in the urine (pyuria) in the first bottle indicates anterior urethritis; bacteria in the urine in the second bottle indicates bladder infection; bacteria in the third bottle indicates prostatitis.

• Signs and symptoms of aortic stenosis include a loud, rough systolic murmur over the aortic area, exertional dyspnea, fatigue, angina pectoris, arrhythmias, low blood pressure, and emboli.

• Elective surgery is primarily a matter of choice. It is not essential to the patient's survival, but it may improve the patient's health, comfort, or self-esteem.

• Required surgery is recommended by the physician. It may be delayed but is inevitable.

• Urgent surgery must be performed within 24 to 48 hours.

• Emergency surgery must be performed immediately.

• Nitrazine paper is used to test urine pH.

• Drug administration is a dependent activity. The nurse can administer or withhold a drug only with the physician's permission.

- About 85% of arterial emboli originate in the heart chambers.

- Pulmonary embolism usually results from thrombi dislodged from the leg veins.

- The average weight gain during a normal pregnancy is 25 to 30 lb (11 to 13.6 kg) total. The patient normally gains 2 to 5 lb (0.9 to 2.3 kg) during the first trimester and slightly less than 1 lb (0.45 kg) per week during the last two trimesters.

- The nurse should not give false assurance to a patient.

- Neonatal jaundice in the first 24 hours after birth is sign of erythroblastosis fetalis.

- A classic difference between placenta previa and abruptio placentae is the degree of pain; abruptio placentae produces more pain.

- After receiving preoperative medication, a patient is not competent to sign an informed consent form.

- The conscious interpretation of pain occurs in the cerebral cortex.

- The dressing on a donor skin graft site should not be disturbed to avoid interfering with new cell growth.

- A sequela is any abnormal condition that follows and is the result of a disease, treatment, or injury.

- Patient care during sickle cell crisis includes bed rest, oxygen therapy, analgesics as prescribed, I.V. fluid monitoring, and thorough documentation of fluid intake and output.

- Reactive depression is a response to a specific life event.

- A patient with an ileal conduit should maintain a daily fluid intake of 2,000 ml.

- The lower central incisors erupt first in an infant.

- In a closed chest drainage system, continuous bubbling in the water seal chamber or bottle indicates a leak.

- Palpitation is a sensation of heart pounding or racing associated with normal emotional responses and certain heart disorders.

- Fat embolism is likely to occur within the first 24 hours after a long bone fracture.

- Footdrop can occur in a patient with a pelvic fracture because of peroneal nerve compression against the head of the fibula.

- To promote venous return after an amputation, the nurse should wrap an elastic (Ace) bandage around the distal end of the stump.

- Because a major role of the placenta is to function as a fetal lung, any condition that interrupts normal blood flow to or from the placenta will increase fetal $PaCO_2$ and decrease fetal pH.

- The oxytocin challenge test determines if the fetus can tolerate uterine contractions. A positive test result suggests the need for cesarean delivery.

- Precipitate labor lasts for only 3 hours and ends with delivery of the neonate.

- Methylergonovine maleate (Methergine) is an oxytocic agent used to prevent and treat postpartal hemorrhage caused by uterine atony or subinvolution.

- As emergency treatment for excessive uterine bleeding, 0.2 mg of methylergonovine maleate (Methergine) is injected I.V. over 1 minute while the patient's blood pressure and uterine contractions are monitored.

- If a child with a febrile illness is schedule for an immunization, the immunization should be postponed.

- Toilet training should begin when a child shows signs of readiness, such as staying dry for 2 hours or more and verbalizing the urge to urinate.

- Most toddlers develop daytime bladder and bowel control between ages 2 and 3. (Failure to achieve toilet training by age 5 usually does not indicate pathology.)

- Projection is the unconscious assigning of a thought, feeling, or action to someone or something else.

- Sublimation is the channeling of unacceptable impulses into socially acceptable behavior.

- Repression is an unconscious defense mechanism whereby unacceptable or painful thoughts, impulses, memories, or feelings are pushed from the consciousness or forgotten.

- The most common administration route for epinephrine is subcutaneous.

- Hypochondriasis is morbid anxiety about one's health associated with various symptoms not caused by organic disease.

- Denial is a refusal to acknowledge feelings, thoughts, desires, impulses, or external facts that are consciously intolerable.

- Reaction formation is the avoidance of anxiety through behavior and attitudes that are the opposite of repressed impulses and drives.

- Displacement is the transfer of unacceptable feelings to a more acceptable object.

- Regression is a retreat to an earlier developmental stage.

- The nurse should use Fowler's position for a patient with abdominal pain caused by appendicitis.

- The nurse should not give analgesics to a patient with abdominal pain caused by appendicitis because these drugs may mask the pain that accompanies a ruptured appendix.

- As a last-ditch effort, a barbiturate coma may be induced to reverse unrelenting increased intracranial pressure (ICP), which is defined as acute ICP above 40 mm Hg, persistent ICP elevation above 20 mm Hg, or rapidly deteriorating neurologic status.

- The primary signs and symptoms of epiglottitis are progressive difficulty in swallowing and a high temperature.

- Salivation is the first step in starch digestion.

- Braxton-Hicks contractions usually are felt in the abdomen and do not cause cervical change, whereas true labor contractions are felt in the front of the abdomen and back and lead to progressive cervical dilatation and effacement.

- The average birth weight of neonates born to mothers who smoke is 6 oz (170 g) less than that of neonates born to nonsmoking mothers.

- When performing CPR on an infant, the rescuer should compress the sternum ½" to 1" (1.3 to 2.5 cm).

- A patient who has a pacemaker should measure the pulse before rising in the morning, notify the physician if the pulse rate exceeds 140 beats/minute, obtain a medical identification card and bracelet, and resume normal activities, including sexual activity.

- Ventricular septal defect occurs because the septum between the left and right ventricles fails to close during the 8th week of gestation.

- Transverse colostomy or loop colostomy is a temporary procedure to divert the fecal stream in a patient with acute intestinal obstruction.

- According to Erikson, an older adult (age 65 or older) is in the developmental stage of integrity versus despair.

- Family therapy focuses on the family as a whole rather than the individual. Its major objective is to reestablish rational communication between family members.

- Conversion reaction is the unconscious transformation of emotions into physical manifestations.

- Normal values for erythrocyte sedimentation rate range from 0 to 15 mm/hr for men under age 50 and from 0 to 20 mm/hr for women under age 50.

- A CPK-MB level that is more than 5% of total CPK or more than 10 units/liter suggests an MI.

- Culdoscopy is visualization of the pelvic organs through the posterior vaginal fornix.

- Propranolol (Inderal) blocks sympathetic nerve stimuli that increase cardiac work during exercise or stress, which reduces heart rate, blood pressure, and myocardial oxygen consumption.

- After an MI, ECG changes (ST-segment elevation, T-wave inversion, and Q-wave enlargement) usually appear in the first 24 hours but may appear in 5 to 6 days.

- Cardiogenic shock is manifested by systolic blood pressure below 80 mm Hg, gray skin, diaphoresis, cyanosis, weak pulse rate, tachycardia or bradycardia, and oliguria of less than 30 ml of urine per hour.

- A patient on a low-sodium diet should not eat such foods as cottage cheese, fish, canned beans, chuck steak, chocolate pudding, Italian salad dressing, dill pickles, and beef broth.

- High-potassium foods include dried prunes, watermelon (15.3 mEq/portion), dried lima beans (14.5 mEq/portion), soybeans, bananas, and oranges.

- A nurse may clarify a physician's explanation to a patient about an operation or a procedure but must refer questions about informed consent to the physician.

- When caring for a hostile or angry patient, the nurse should attempt to remain calm, listen without showing disapproval, speak in a firm, quiet voice, and use short sentences.

- A sick or injured child with limited communication skills may be able to express feelings or concerns by drawing a picture with crayons or markers.

- When obtaining a health history from an acutely ill or agitated patient, the nurse should limit questions to those that provide necessary information.

- Before taking an oral temperature, the nurse should ensure that the patient has not consumed anything cold or hot or smoked a cigarette for at least 15 minutes.

- The nurse should not use the thumb to take a patient's pulse because the thumb has a pulse of its own and may be confused with the patient's pulse.

- An inspiration and an expiration count as one respiration.

- Kussmaul's respirations are faster and deeper than normal respirations and occur without pauses.

- Cheyne-Stokes respirations are characterized by alternating periods of apnea and deep, rapid breathing.

- Hyperventilation can result from an increased frequency of breathing, an increased tidal volume, or both.

- Apnea is the absence of spontaneous respirations.

- Before a thyroidectomy, a patient may receive potassium iodide (SSKI), antithyroid drugs, and propranolol (Inderal) to prevent thyroid storm during surgery.

- Normal respirations are known as *eupnea.*

- During a blood pressure measurement, the patient should rest the arm against a surface because using muscle strength to hold up the arm may raise the blood pressure.

- Major unalterable risk factors for coronary artery disease include heredity, sex, race, and age.

- The nurse should teach a pregnant vegetarian to obtain protein from alternate sources, such as nuts, soybeans, and legumes.

- Inspection is the most frequently used assessment technique.

- The nurse should instruct a pregnant patient to take only prescribed prenatal vitamins because over-the-counter (OTC) megavitamins may harm the fetus.

- High-sodium foods can cause fluid retention, especially in pregnant patients.

- A pregnant patient can avoid constipation and hemorrhoids by adding fiber to her diet.

- The normal life span of RBCs (erythrocytes) is 110 to 120 days.

- Ritualism and negativism are typical toddler behaviors. They occur during the developmental stage identified by Erikson as autonomy versus shame and doubt.

- Accidents are the leading cause of death in children and usually are age-related—for example, toddlers are injured in falls and teenagers are injured in sports.

- Urinary tract infections are more common in girls and women than in boys and men because the shorter urethra in the female urinary tract makes the bladder more accessible to bacteria, especially *Escherichia coli.*

- Visual acuity of 20/100 means that the patient sees at 20 ft (6 m) what a person with normal vision sees at 100 ft (30 m).

- According to Freud, the oral stage occurs between birth and age 18 months.

- Penicillin should be administered 1 to 2 hours before meals or 2 to 3 hours after meals because food may interfere with the drug's absorption.

- For an infant, the nurse should start an I.V. line in a peripheral vein or a vein in the temporal region.

- Mild reactions to local anesthetics may include palpitations, tinnitus, vertigo, apprehension, confusion, and a metallic taste in the mouth.

- When administering an oral medication to a toddler, the nurse should have the child place the medication on the back of the tongue and swallow it with fruit juice or water.

- Family members of an elderly person in a long-term care facility should transfer some personal items (such as photographs, a favorite chair, and knickknacks) to the person's room to provide a homey atmosphere.

- About 22% of cardiac output goes to the kidneys.

- To ensure accurate CVP readings, the nurse should place the manometer or transducer level with the phlebostatic axis.

- A patient who has lost 2,000 to 2,500 ml of blood will have a pulse rate of 140 beats/minute (or higher), display a systolic blood pressure of 50 to 60 mm Hg, and appear confused and lethargic.

- Arterial bleeding is bright red, flows rapidly, and (because it is pumped directly from the heart) spurts with each heartbeat.

- Venous blood is dark red and tends to ooze from a wound.

• Orthostatic blood pressure is taken with the patient in the supine, sitting, and standing positions and with 1 minute between each reading. A 10-mm Hg decrease in blood pressure or a pulse rate increase of 10 beats/minute suggests volume depletion.

• Pulsus alternans is a regular pulse rhythm with alternation of weak and strong beats. It occurs in ventricular enlargement because the stroke volume varies with each heartbeat.

• Medical antishock trousers (MAST) should be used cautiously with pregnant women and patients with head injuries.

• After a patient's circulating volume has been restored, the nurse should remove the MAST suit gradually, starting with the abdominal chamber and followed by each leg. Removal should be done under a physician's supervision.

• Most hemolytic transfusion reactions associated with ABO mismatching stem from identification number errors.

• Circumstantiality is a disturbance in associate thought and speech patterns in which a patient gives unnecessary, minute details and digresses into inappropriate thoughts, which delay communication of central ideas or goal achievement.

• Warming of blood above 107° F (41.6° C) can cause hemolysis.

• Cardiac output is the amount of blood ejected from the heart each minute and is expressed in liters per minute.

• Stroke volume is the volume of blood ejected from the heart during systole.

• TPN solution contains dextrose, amino acids, and additives such as electrolytes, minerals, and vitamins.

• The most common type of neurogenic shock is spinal shock. It usually occurs 30 to 60 minutes after a spinal cord injury.

- After a spinal cord injury, peristalsis stops within 24 hours and usually returns within 3 to 4 days.

- Toxic shock syndrome is manifested by a temperature of at least 102º F (38.8º C), an erythematous rash, and systolic blood pressure below 90 mm Hg. From 1 to 2 weeks after the onset of these signs, desquamation (especially on the palms and soles) occurs.

- The signs and symptoms of anaphylaxis commonly are caused by histamine release.

- The most common cause of septic shock is gram-negative bacteria, such as *Escherichia coli, Klebsiella pneumonia,* and *Pseudomonas* organisms.

- Bruits are vascular sounds that resemble heart murmurs and result from turbulent blood flow through a diseased or partially obstructed artery.

- Urine pH normally ranges from 4.5 to 8.0.

- Urine pH greater than 8.0 can result from a urinary tract infection, high-alkali diet, or systemic alkalosis.

- Urine pH less than 4.5 may indicate a high-protein diet, fever, or metabolic acidosis.

- Before a percutaneous renal biopsy, the patient should be placed on a firm surface and positioned on the abdomen with a sandbag under the abdomen to stabilize the kidneys.

- Nephrotic syndrome is characterized by marked proteinuria, hypoalbuminemia, mild to severe dependent edema, and ascites.

- Underwater exercise is a form of therapy performed in a Hubbard tank.

- Laboratory findings in nephrotic syndrome include proteinuria, hypoalbuminemia, and hyperlipidemia.

• Most women with trichomoniasis have a malodorous, frothy, greenish gray vaginal discharge; other women may have no signs or symptoms.

• Voiding cystourethrography may be done to detect bladder and urethral abnormalities. In this test, contrast medium is instilled by gentle syringe pressure through a urethral catheter, and overhead X-ray films are taken to visualize bladder filling and excretion.

• Cystourethrography may be done to help identify the cause of urinary tract infections, congenital anomalies, and incontinence. It also is used to assess for prostate lobe hypertrophy in men.

• Herpes simplex, characterized by recurrent episodes of blisters on the skin and mucous membrane, has two variations. In type I, the blisters appear in the nasolabial region; in type II, they appear on the genitals, anus, buttocks, and thighs.

• Most patients with *Chlamydia trachomatis* infection are asymptomatic, but some develop an inflamed urethral meatus, dysuria, and urinary urgency and frequency.

• The hypothalamus regulates the autonomic nervous system and endocrine functions.

• If a pregnant patient develops late deceleration (a sign of fetal hypoxia), the nurse should instruct her to lay on her side and should notify the physician. (The side-lying position removes pressure on the inferior vena cava.)

• Oxytocin (Pitocin) promotes lactation and uterine contractions.

• The upper respiratory tract warms and humidifies inspired air and plays a role in taste, smell, and mastication.

• A patient whose chest excursion is less than normal (3" to 6" [7.5 to 15 cm]) must use accessory muscles to breathe.

• Signs of accessory muscle use include shoulder elevation, intercostal muscle retraction, and scalene and sternocleidomastoid muscle use during respiration.

• Lanugo covers the fetus's body until about 20 weeks' gestation. Then it begins to disappear from the face, trunk, arms, and legs, in that order.

• Although a cleft palate can be repaired at any time, the optimal time for corrective surgery is before the child begins speaking and learns faulty speech habits.

• In a neonate, hypoglycemia is manifested by temperature instability, hypotonia, jitteriness, and seizures. Premature, postmature, small-for-gestational-age, and large-for-gestational-age neonates are prone to this disorder.

• An infant with a gastrostomy tube should receive a pacifier during feeding to allow normal sucking activity and satisfy oral needs.

• Signs and symptoms of toxicity from thyroid replacement therapy include rapid pulse rate, diaphoresis, irritability, weight loss, dysuria, and sleep disturbance.

• The most common allergic reaction to penicillin is a rash.

• An early sign of aspirin toxicity is deep, rapid respirations.

• The most serious and irreversible consequence of lead poisoning is mental retardation, which results from neurologic damage.

• Treatment of Legg-Calve-Perthes disease consists of restricting weight bearing and using such devices as an abduction brace or a harness sling to protect the affected joint while revascularization and bone healing occur.

• Gastroesophageal reflux scanning uses less radiation and is a more sensitive test than conventional barium swallow testing.

- Legg-Calve-Perthes disease (also known as coxa plana) is manifested in aseptic necrosis of the head of the femur.

- In developing a diet for a patient with a peptic ulcer, the nurse should remember this guideline: The type of diet is less important than including foods in the diet that the patient can tolerate.

- A patient with a colostomy needs to establish an irrigation schedule so that regular emptying of the bowel occurs without stomal discharge between irrigations.

- Idea of reference is an incorrect belief that the statements or actions of others are related to oneself.

- When using rotating tourniquets, the nurse should not restrict the blood supply to an arm or a leg for more than 45 minutes at a time.

- A patient with diabetes should eat high-fiber foods because they blunt the rise in glucose that normally follows a meal.

- Jugular vein distention occurs in CHF because the left ventricle cannot empty the heart of blood as fast as blood enters from the right ventricle, resulting in congestion in the entire venous system.

- When using axillary crutches, the patient's palms should bear the brunt of the weight.

- The leading causes of blindness in the United States are diabetes mellitus and glaucoma.

- After a thyroidectomy, the patient should remain in semi-Fowler's position with the head neither hyperextended nor hyperflexed to avoid pressure on the suture line.

- Premenstrual syndrome may cause abdominal distention, engorged and painful breasts, backache, headache, nervousness, irritability, restlessness, and tremors.

- Treatment of dehiscence (pathologic opening of a wound) consists of covering the wound with a moist sterile dressing and notifying the physician.

- When a patient has a radical mastectomy, the ovaries also may be removed because they are a source of estrogen, which stimulates tumor growth.

- Atropine sulfate blocks the effects of acetylcholine, thereby obstructing its vagal effects on the sinoatrial node and increasing heart rate.

- Activities of daily living include eating, bathing, dressing, grooming, toileting, and interacting socially.

- Salicylates, particularly aspirin, are the treatment of choice in rheumatoid arthritis because they decrease inflammation and relieve joint pain.

- Deep, intense pain that usually worsens at night and is unrelated to movement suggests bone pain.

- Pain that follows prolonged or excessive exercise and subsides with rest suggests muscle pain.

- Normal gait has two phases: the stance phase, in which the patient's foot rests on the ground, and the swing phase, in which the patient's foot moves forward.

- The major hemodynamic changes associated with cardio-genic shock are decreased left ventricular function and decreased cardiac output.

- Before thyroidectomy, the patient should be advised that he may experience hoarseness or loss of the voice for several days after surgery.

- Acceptable adverse effects of long-term steroid use include weight gain, acne, headaches, fatigue, and increased urine retention.

• Unacceptable adverse effects of long-term steroid use are dizziness on rising, nausea, vomiting, thirst, and pain.

• After a craniotomy, nursing care includes maintaining normal ICP, maintaining cerebral perfusion pressure, and preventing injury related to cerebral and cellular ischemia.

• Every day, neonates typically need to consume 50 to 55 calories per pound of body weight.

• Folic acid and vitamin B_{12} are essential for nucleoprotein synthesis and RBC maturation.

• Immediately after intracranial surgery, nursing care includes not giving the patient anything by mouth until gag and cough reflexes return, elevating the head of the bed 30 degrees after the patient regains consciousness, monitoring vital signs and assessing level of consciousness for signs of increasing ICP, and giving analgesics that do not mask the patient's level of consciousness.

• Chest physiotherapy includes postural drainage, chest percussion and vibration, coughing, and deep-breathing exercises.

• The nurse should encourage parents to communicate with their hearing-impaired child through mime, gestures, and body language.

• Kawasaki disease is characterized by a high temperature for 5 or more days, strawberry tongue, red and dry lips, cervical lymphadenopathy, carditis, hand edema, rash on the soles or palms, and bilateral congestion of the ocular conjunctivae.

• Cushing's syndrome results from excessive levels of adrenocortical hormones and is manifested by fat pads on the face (moon face) and over the upper back (buffalo hump), acne, mood swings, hirsutism, amenorrhea, and decreased libido.

- When discontinuing long-term prednisone (Deltasone) therapy, the nurse should taper the dose slowly to allow for monitoring of disease flare-ups and for the return of hypothalamic-pituitary-adrenal function.

- Pulsus paradoxus (a pulse that becomes weak during inspiration and strong during expiration) may be a sign of cardiac tamponade.

- Substances expelled through portals of exit include saliva, mucus, feces, urine, vomitus, blood, and vaginal and penile discharge.

- A microorganism may be transmitted directly by contact with an infected body or droplets or indirectly by contact with contaminated air, soil, water, or fluids.

- A postmenopausal woman receiving estrogen therapy is at increased risk of developing gallbladder disease.

- The approximate oxygen concentrations delivered by nasal cannula are as follows: 1 liter = 24%, 2 liters = 28%, 3 liters = 32%, 4 liters = 36%, and 5 liters = 40%.

- Because oxytocin (Pitocin) stimulates powerful uterine contractions during labor, it must be administered under close observation to help prevent maternal and fetal distress.

- Cardinal features of diabetes insipidus include polydipsia (excessive thirst) and polyuria (increased urination to 5 liters/24 hours).

- A patient with low specific gravity (1.001 to 1.005) may have an increased desire for cold water.

- Diabetic coma can occur when the blood glucose level drops below 60 mg/dl.

- For a patient with CHF, the nurse should elevate the head of the bed 8" to 12" (20 to 30 cm), provide a bedside commode, and administer digitalis and diuretics as prescribed.

- Group therapy provides an opportunity for each group member to examine interactions, learn and practice successful interpersonal communication skills, and explore emotional conflicts.

- The primary reason for treating streptococcal sore throat with antibiotics is to protect the heart valves and prevent rheumatic fever.

- A patient with a nasal fracture may lose consciousness during reduction.

- Hoarseness may be the first sign of laryngeal cancer.

- The lungs, colon, and rectum are among the most common cancer sites.

- The most common preoperative problem in elderly patients is lower-than-normal total blood volume.

- Mannitol (Osmitrol), an osmotic diuretic, is administered to reduce intraocular or intracranial pressure.

- When CVA is suspected, the nurse should place the patient on the affected side to promote lung expansion on the unaffected side.

- For a patient who has had chest surgery, the nurse should recommend sitting upright and performing deep-breathing and coughing exercises. These actions promote lung expansion, secretion removal, and optimal pulmonary functioning.

- During fetal heart monitoring, variable deceleration indicates umbilical cord compression or prolapse.

- During every sleep cycle, the sleeper passes through four stages of nonrapid-eye-movement (NREM) sleep and one stage of rapid-eye-movement (REM) sleep.

- The phases of mitosis are prophase, metaphase, anaphase, and telophase.

- Korsakoff's syndrome is believed to be a chronic form of Wernicke's encephalopathy marked by hallucinations, confabulation, amnesia, and disturbances of orientation.

- A patient taking calcifediol (Calderol) should avoid concomitant use of preparations that contain vitamin D.

- A patient should begin and end a 24-hour urine collection period with an empty bladder. (For example, if the physician orders urine to be collected from 0800 Thursday to 0800 Friday, the urine voided at 0800 Thursday should be discarded and the urine voided at 0800 Friday should be retained.)

- In a patient receiving digoxin (Lanoxin), a low potassium level increases the risk of digitalis toxicity.

- BUN values normally range from 10 to 20 mg/dl.

- Flurazepam (Dalmane) toxicity is manifested by confusion, hallucinations, and ataxia.

- A silent MI is one that produces no symptoms.

- Adverse reactions to verapamil (Isoptin) include dizziness, headache, constipation, hypotension, and atrioventricular conduction disturbances. The drug also may increase the serum digoxin level.

- When a rectal tube is used to relieve flatulence or enhance peristalsis, it should be inserted for no more than 20 minutes.

- Yellowish green discharge on a wound dressing indicates infection and should be cultured.

- Sickle cell crisis can cause severe abdominal, thoracic, muscular, and bone pain along with painful swelling of soft tissue in the hands and feet.

- Oral candidiasis (thrush) is characterized by cream-colored or bluish white patches on the oral mucous membrane.

- Treatment for a patient with cystic fibrosis may include drug therapy; exercises to improve breathing and posture and facilitate mobilization of pulmonary secretions; a high-salt diet; and pancreatic enzyme supplements.

- After surgical reconstruction of an imperforate anus and formation of a temporary colostomy, an infant should remain prone with the hips elevated.

- A patient with antisocial personality disorder frequently engages in confrontations with authority figures, such as police, parents, and school officials.

- A patient with paranoid personality disorder exhibits suspicion, hypervigilance, and hostility toward others.

- Child neglect consists of abandonment or failure to provide a safe, secure environment for a child.

- Depression is the most common psychiatric disorder.

- Cytomegalovirus (CMV) is the leading cause of congenital viral infections.

- Most infants with cerebral palsy are long and thin, move asymmetrically, have difficulty feeding, and cry excessively or feebly.

- Pancreatic cancer may cause weight loss, jaundice, and intermittent dull-to-severe epigastric pain.

- Adverse reactions to tricyclic antidepressant drugs include tachycardia, orthostatic hypotension, hypomania, lowered seizure threshold, tremors, weight gain, problems with erections or orgasms, and anxiety.

- The nurse should follow universal precautions in the routine care of all patients.

- Metastasis is the spread of cancer from one organ to another.

- Tocolytic therapy is indicated in premature labor but contraindicated in fetal death, fetal distress, or severe hemorrhage.

- The management of pulmonary edema focuses on opening the airways, supporting ventilation and perfusion, improving cardiac functioning, reducing preload, and reducing patient anxiety.

- Factors that contribute to the death of patients with Alzheimer's disease include infection, malnutrition, and dehydration.

- Hodgkin's disease is characterized by painless, progressive enlargement of cervical lymph nodes and other lymphoid tissue resulting from proliferation of Reed-Sternberg cells, histiocytes, and eosinophils.

- Huntington's disease (chorea) is a hereditary disease characterized by degeneration in the cerebral cortex and basal ganglia.

- A patient with Huntington's disease may exhibit suicidal ideation.

- At discharge, an amputee should be able to demonstrate proper stump care and perform stump-toughening exercises.

- Acute tubular necrosis is the most common cause of acute renal failure.

- Common complications of ice water lavage are vomiting and aspiration.

- Foods high in vitamin D include fortified milk, fish, liver, liver oil, herring, and egg yolk.

- Through ultrasonography, the biophysical profile assesses fetal well-being by measuring fetal breathing movements, gross body movements, fetal tone, reactive FHR (nonstress test), and qualitative amniotic fluid volume.

- For a pelvic examination, the patient should be in the lithotomy position with her buttocks extending 2½" (6.4 cm) past the end of the examination table.

- If a patient cannot assume a lithotomy position, she may lay on her left side.

- A male examiner should have a female assistant present during a vaginal examination for the patient's emotional comfort and the examiner's legal protection.

- Cervical secretions are clear and stretchy before ovulation and white and opaque after ovulation. They normally are odorless and do not irritate the mucosa.

- A neonate whose mother has diabetes should be assessed for hyperinsulinism.

- Epigastric pain is a late symptom in a patient with preeclampsia and requires immediate medical intervention.

- After a stillbirth, the mother should be allowed to hold the neonate to help her come to terms with the death.

- The concept of object permanence develops between ages 6 and 8 months.

- A child begins to understand cause-and-effect relations at age 2, during the sensorimotor stage.

- Attention deficit disorder and learning disabilities are more common among boys than girls.

- A patient with an ileostomy should not eat corn because it may obstruct the pouch opening.

- *Molding* describes the process by which the fetal head changes shape to facilitate movement through the birth canal.

- Liver dysfunction affects the metabolism of certain drugs.

- If a patient receives a pudendal block before delivery, the nurse should monitor the patient's blood pressure closely.

- If a patient suddenly becomes hypotensive during labor, the nurse should increase the infusion rate of I.V. fluids, as prescribed.

- The best technique for assessing jaundice in a neonate is to blanch the skin on the forehead.

- During fetal heart monitoring, early deceleration is caused by head compression during labor.

- After the placenta is delivered, the nurse may add oxytocin (Pitocin) to the patient's I.V. solution as prescribed to promote postpartal evacuation of the uterus and stimulate lactation.

- Pica is a craving to eat nonfood items, such as dirt, crayons, chalk, glue, starch, or hair. It may occur during pregnancy and can endanger the fetus.

- A pregnant patient should take folic acid because this nutrient is required for rapid cell division.

- Edema that accompanies burns and malnutrition is caused by decreased capillary osmotic pressure.

- Hyponatremia is most likely to occur as a complication of nasogastric suctioning.

- For a man who suffers complete spinal cord separation at S4, erection and ejaculation are not possible.

- The early signs of pulmonary edema—dyspnea on exertion and coughing—reflect interstitial fluid accumulation and diminished ventilation and alveolar perfusion.

- Methylprednisolone sodium succinate (Solu-Medrol) is a first-line drug used to control edema after spinal cord trauma.

- For the patient who is recovering from an intracranial bleed, the nurse should maintain a quiet, restful environment for the first few days.

- The patient taking clomiphene citrate (Clomid) to induce ovulation should be informed of the possibility of multiple births with this drug.

- Neurosyphilis is associated with widespread CNS damage, including general paresis, personality changes, slapping gait, and blindness.

- A woman who has sustained a spinal cord injury can still become pregnant.

- In a patient who has had a CVA, the most serious complication is increasing ICP.

- If needed, cervical suturing usually is done between 14 and 18 weeks' gestation to reinforce an incompetent cervix and maintain pregnancy. Such suturing typically is removed by 35 weeks' gestation.

- A patient with an intracranial hemorrhage should undergo arteriography to determine the site of the bleeding.

- Factors that affect drug action include absorption, distribution, metabolism, and excretion.

- During the first trimester, a pregnant women should avoid all medications unless doing so would adversely affect her health.

- Before prescribing a medication for a woman of childbearing age, the prescriber should ask for the date of her last menstrual period and ask if she may be pregnant.

- Most medications a breast-feeding mother takes appear in breast milk.

- Acidosis may cause insulin resistance.

- A patient with G6PD deficiency may develop acute hemolytic anemia when given a sulfonamide.

- The Food and Drug Administration has established five categories of drugs based on their potential for causing birth defects: A - No evidence of risk; B - No risk found in animals, but no studies have been done in women; C - Animal studies have shown an adverse effect, but the drug may be beneficial to women despite the potential risk; D - Evidence of risk, but its benefits may outweigh its risks; and X - Fetal anomalies noted, and the risks clearly outweigh the potential benefits.

- The five basic activities of the digestive system include ingestion, movement of food, digestion, absorption, and defecation.

- The nurse should use the bell of the stethoscope to listen for venous hums and murmurs.

- In the chief complaint section of the health record, the nurse can record the patient's needs and concerns in his or her own words.

- Signs and symptoms of acute pancreatitis include epigastric pain, vomiting, discolored flank (Grey Turner's sign), low-grade fever, tachycardia, and hypotension.

- A patient with a gastric ulcer may complain of gnawing or burning epigastric pain.

- The nurse can assess a patient's general knowledge by asking such questions as "Who is the President of the United States?"

- To test the first cranial nerve (olfactory nerve), the nurse should ask the patient to close the eyes, occlude one nostril, and identify a nonirritating substance (such as peppermint or cinnamon) by smell. Then the nurse should repeat the test with the patient's other nostril occluded.

- Salk and Sabin introduced the oral polio vaccine.

- A patient with a disease of the cerebellum or posterior column displays an ataxic gait, characterized by staggering, unsteadiness, and an inability to remain steady when standing with the feet together.

- Improved outcomes for trauma patients are directly related to early resuscitation, aggressive management of shock, and appropriate definitive care.

- To check for cerebrospinal fluid leakage, the nurse should inspect the patient's nose and ears. If the patient can sit up, the nurse should observe for leakage as the patient leans forward.

- For a child suspected of having Reye's syndrome, the nurse should ask the parents if the child received aspirin during the current or a recent illness.

- "Locked-in" syndrome is complete paralysis caused by brain stem damage; only the eyes can be moved voluntarily.

- Neck dissection, the surgical removal of the cervical lymph nodes, is performed to prevent the spread of malignant head and neck tumors.

- A patient with cholecystitis typically complains of right epigastric pain, nausea, and vomiting, especially after eating a heavy meal.

- A patient with a ruptured ectopic pregnancy commonly has sharp lower abdominal pain with spotting and cramping and may experience abdominal rigidity, rapid and shallow respirations, tachycardia, and shock.

- A patient on prednisone or another steroid should not stop taking the medication abruptly.

- Serum calcium levels normally range from 4.5 to 5.5 mEq/liter.

- Suppressor T cells regulate overall immune response.

- Serum levels of aspartate aminotransferase (AST, formerly serum glutamic-oxaloacetic transaminase) and serum alanine aminotransferase (ALT, formerly serum glutamic-pyruvic transaminase) reveal whether the liver is adequately detoxifying medications.

- Serum sodium levels normally range from 135 to 145 mEq/liter.

- Serum potassium levels normally range from 3.5 to 5.0 mEq/liter.

- A patient taking prednisone (Deltasone) should consume a salt-restricted diet that is rich in potassium and protein.

- A nurse who performs continuous ambulatory peritoneal dialysis must use sterile technique when caring for the catheter, send a peritoneal fluid sample for culture and sensitivity testing every 24 hours, and report signs of infection and fluid imbalance.

- The Minnesota Multiphasic Personality Inventory consists of 550 statements for the subject to interpret. It assesses personality and detects disorders, such as depression and schizophrenia, in adolescents and adults.

- TORCH infections include toxoplasmosis, other diseases (chlamydia, group B beta-hemolytic streptococcus, syphilis, and varicella zoster), rubella, cytomegalovirus, and herpesvirus. Because these infections can harm an embryo or a fetus, the nurse assesses for these in a pregnant patient or one considering pregnancy.

- An infant infected with HIV during gestation typically begins to show signs and symptoms, such as fever, adenopathy, rash, diarrhea, and failure to thrive, between ages 2 and 4 months.

- When working with AIDS patients, the nurse should wear a mask only if the possibility exists that blood or some other body fluid will splash on the face.

- HIV-infected blood spills should be cleaned up with a 1:10 solution of sodium hypochlorite 5.25% (household bleach).

- Raynaud's phenomenon is intermittent ischemic attacks in the fingers or toes marked by severe pallor and, sometimes, paresthesia and pain.

- Intussusception (prolapse of one bowel segment into the lumen of another) causes the sudden onset of epigastric pain, sausage-shaped abdominal swelling, passage of mucus and blood through the rectum, shock, and hypotension.

- The mechanics of delivery are engagement, descent and flexion, internal rotation, extension, external rotation, restitution, and expulsion.

- Bence Jones protein occurs almost exclusively in the urine of patients with multiple myeloma.

- Gaucher's disease is an autosomal disorder characterized by abnormal accumulation of glucocerebrosides (lipid substances that contain a glucose sugar) in monocytes and macrocytes. It occurs in three forms: type I is the adult form; type II, the infantile form; and type III, the juvenile form.

- A patient with colon obstruction may develop lower abdominal pain, constipation, increasing distention, and vomiting.

- A medication is double strength if D.S. follows its name.

- Colchicine (Colsalide) relieves inflammation and is used to treat gout.

- Some people develop hyperuricemia because they cannot metabolize and excrete purines normally.

- A normal sperm count ranges from 20 to 150 million/ml.

- Organic brain syndrome is the most common form of mental illness in elderly patients.

• Clues to physical abuse of a child include inconsistent stories from parents about how the injuries occurred, lack of permission for the child to speak, wounds that do not match the mechanism of injury or are at different stages of healing, and unexplained injuries.

• A first-degree burn involves the stratum corneum layer of the epidermis and is manifested as pain and redness.

• Sheehan's syndrome is hypopituitarism caused by a pituitary infarct after postpartal shock and hemorrhage.

• When caring for a patient with an asthma attack, the nurse should place the patient in Fowler's or semi-Fowler's position.

• Among elderly patients, the incidence of noncompliance with prescribed drug therapy is high because many elderly patients have diminished visual acuity, hearing loss, or forgetfulness or need to take multiple drugs.

• Tuberculosis is a reportable communicable disease caused by infection with *Mycobacterium tuberculosis* (an acid-fast bacillus).

• For right-sided cardiac catheterization, the physician passes a multilumen catheter through the superior or inferior vena cava.

• A probable sign of pregnancy, McDonald's sign is characterized by an ease in flexing the body of the uterus against the cervix.

• Amenorrhea is not a conclusive sign of pregnancy.

• A pregnant woman's partner should avoid introducing air into the vagina during oral sex because of the possibility of air embolism.

• The presence of human chorionic gonadotropin in the blood or urine is a probable sign of pregnancy.

- Radiography usually is not used in a pregnant patient because it may harm the developing fetus. However, if radiography is essential, it should be performed only after 36 weeks' gestation.

- After a fracture, bone healing occurs in these stages: hematoma formation, cellular proliferation and callus formation, and ossification and remodeling.

- In a pregnant patient, membrane rupture or vaginal bleeding contraindicates intercourse.

- A patient scheduled for positron emission tomography should avoid alcohol, tobacco, and caffeine for 24 hours before the test.

- Milia may occur as pinpoint spots over a neonate's nose.

- In CVA, decreased oxygen destroys brain cells.

- A contraction's duration is timed from the moment the uterus tightens until it relaxes.

- A person with an IQ of less than 20 is profoundly retarded and considered a total-care patient.

- The union of a male and a female gamete produces a zygote, which divides into the fertilized ovum.

- A patient with glaucoma should not receive atropine sulfate because this drug increases intraocular pressure.

- The nurse should instruct a hyperventilating patient to rebreathe into a paper bag.

- The first menstrual flow is called menarche and may be anovulatory (infertile).

- The pons is located above the medulla and consists of white matter (sensory and motor tracts) and gray matter (reflex centers).

- During IPPB, the patient should bite down on the mouth-piece, breathe normally, and let the machine do the work. After inspiration, the patient should hold the breath for 3 to 4 seconds and exhale completely through the mouthpiece.

- The autonomic nervous system controls the smooth muscles.

- A patient who sits in a wheelchair for a long time may develop flexion contractures of the hips.

- Nystagmus is rapid horizontal or rotating eye movement.

- After myelography, a patient should remain recumbent for 24 hours.

- The treatment for sprains and strains consists of immediately applying ice and elevating the arm or leg above heart level.

- An anticholinesterase agent should not be prescribed for a patient taking morphine because it can potentiate the effect of morphine and cause respiratory depression.

- The primary purpose of play therapy for a hospitalized child is to allow the expression of feelings and frustrations.

- Reframing is a therapeutic technique used with depressed patients to help them to view a situation in alternate ways.

- A correctly written patient goal expresses the desired patient behavior, criteria for measurement, time frame for achievement, and conditions under which the behavior will occur. It is developed in collaboration with the patient.

- Percussion produces five basic notes: tympany (loud intensity, as heard over a gastric air bubble or puffed out cheek), hyperresonance (very loud, as heard over an emphysematous lung), resonance (loud, as heard over a normal lung), dullness (medium intensity, as heard over the liver or other solid organ), and flatness (soft, as heard over the thigh).

- Myopia is nearsightedness; hyperopia and presbyopia are two types of farsightedness.

- The optic disk is yellowish pink and circular with a distinct border.

- The watch-tick test evaluates a person's ability to hear high-frequency sounds. It is performed by gradually moving a watch away from the ear until the person no longer can hear the ticking; a person with normal hearing can hear the watch 5" (13 cm) away.

- The most effective contraceptive method is one that the woman selects for herself and uses consistently.

- Weber's test evaluates bone conduction by placing a vibrating tuning fork on top of the patient's head at midline. The patient should perceive the sound equally in both ears. If the patient has conductive hearing loss, the sound will be heard in (lateralizes to) the ear that has conductive loss.

- The Rinne test evaluates bone conduction by placing a vibrating tuning fork on the mastoid process of the temporal bone, and air conduction by holding the vibrating tuning fork ½" (1.3 cm) from the external auditory meatus until it is no longer heard.

- A primary disability results from a pathologic process; a secondary disability, from inactivity.

- After an amputation, the stump may shrink because of muscle atrophy and decreased subcutaneous fat.

- A patient with rheumatoid arthritis experiences the severest pain in the joint.

- During the umbrella procedure, a treatment for deep vein thrombosis, the surgeon inserts a filter device in the inferior vena cava to trap large emboli before they progress to the lungs.

- After pneumonectomy, the patient should be positioned on the operative side or on the back with the head slightly elevated.

- To reduce the possibility of new emboli formation or expansion, a patient with deep vein thrombosis should receive heparin.

- Atherosclerosis is the most common cause of coronary artery disease and usually involves the aorta and the femoral, coronary, and cerebral arteries.

- Pulmonary embolism is a potentially fatal complication of deep vein thrombosis.

- Chest pain is the most common symptom of pulmonary embolism.

- The nurse should inform a patient taking phenazopyridine hydrochloride (Pyridium) that this medication colors urine orange or red.

- Pneumothorax is a serious complication of central venous line placement; it is caused by inadvertent lung puncture.

- *Pneumocystis carinii* pneumonia normally is not considered contagious because it only affects patients with a suppressed immune system.

- To enhance drug absorption, the patient should take regular erythromycin tablets with a full glass of water 1 hour before or 2 hours after a meal or should take enteric-coated tablets with food. The patient should avoid taking either type of tablets with fruit juice.

- Trismus, a sign of tetanus (lockjaw), is manifested in painful spasms of masticatory muscles, difficulty opening the mouth, neck rigidity and stiffness, and dysphagia.

- Nurses usually are held liable for failing to keep an accurate count of sponges and other devices during surgery.

- The best dietary sources of vitamin B_6 are liver, kidney, pork, soybeans, corn, and whole-grain cereals.

- The nurse should place the patient in an upright position for thoracentesis. If this is not possible, the nurse should position the patient on the unaffected side.

- The nurse should hang a blood bag 3 ft (1 m) above the level of the planned venipuncture site.

- The nurse should place a patient with a closed chest drainage in semi-Fowler's position.

- Iron-rich foods, such as organ meats, nuts, legumes, dried fruit, leafy vegetables, eggs, and whole grains, generally have a low water content.

- If blood is not transfused within 30 minutes, the nurse should return it to the blood bank because the refrigeration facilities on a nursing unit are inadequate for storing blood products.

- Blood that is discolored and contains gas bubbles is contaminated with bacteria and should not be transfused. Fifty percent of patients who receive contaminated blood die.

- For massive, rapid blood transfusions and for exchange transfusions in neonates, blood should be warmed to 98.7° F (37° C).

- A chest tube permits air and fluid drainage from the pleural cavity.

- A hand-held resuscitation bag, such as the Ambu bag, is an inflatable device that can be attached to a face mask or endotracheal or tracheostomy tube; it allows manual delivery of oxygen to the lungs of a patient who cannot breathe independently.

- Mechanical ventilation artificially controls or assists respiration.

- The nurse should encourage a patient with a closed chest drainage system to cough frequently and breathe deeply to help drain the pleural space and expand the lungs.

- Tracheal suction removes secretions from the trachea and bronchi by means of a suction catheter.

- During colostomy irrigation, the irrigation bag should be hung 18" (45 cm) above the stoma.

- The water used for colostomy irrigation should be 100° to 105° F (37.8° to 40.5° C).

- An arterial embolism may cause pain or anesthesia, pallor, coolness, or paralysis in the affected arm or leg.

- Respiratory alkalosis results from conditions that cause hyperventilation and reduce the carbon dioxide level.

- Mineral oil is contraindicated in a patient with appendicitis, acute surgical abdomen, fecal impaction, or intestinal obstruction.

- When using a Y-type administration set to transfuse packed RBCs, the nurse can add 0.9% saline solution to the bag to dilute the RBCs and make them less viscous.

- Autotransfusion is the collection, filtration, and reinfusion of the patient's own blood.

- *Collaboration* refers to joint communication and decision-making between nurses and physicians designed to meet patients' needs by integrating the care regimens of both professions in one comprehensive approach.

- *Bradycardia* refers to a heart rate of fewer than 60 beats/ minute.

- A nursing diagnosis is a statement of a patient's actual or potential health problems that can be resolved, diminished, or otherwise changed by nursing interventions.

- During the assessment phase of the nursing process, the nurse collects and analyzes three types of data: health history, health physical examination, and laboratory and diagnostic test data.

- The patient's health history consists primarily of subjective data—information supplied by the patient.

- The physical examination includes objective data obtained by inspection, palpation, percussion, and auscultation.

- When documenting patient care, the nurse should write legibly, use only standard abbreviations, and sign every entry. The nurse should never destroy or attempt to obliterate documentation or leave vacant lines.

- Factors that affect body temperature include time of day, age, physical activity, phase of menstrual cycle, and pregnancy.

- The most accessible and commonly used artery for measuring a patient's pulse is the radial artery, which is compressed against the radius to take the pulse.

- The normal pulse rate of a resting adult is 60 to 100 beats/minute. The rate is slightly faster in women than in men and much faster in children than in adults.

- Prepared I.V. solutions fall into three general categories: isotonic, hypotonic, and hypertonic. Isotonic solutions possess a solute concentration similar to body fluids; their addition to plasma does not change plasma osmolarity. Hypotonic solutions have a lower osmotic pressure than body fluid; their addition decreases plasma osmolarity. Hypertonic solutions have a higher osmotic pressure than body fluids; their addition increases plasma osmolarity.

- Stress incontinence refers to involuntary urine leakage triggered by a sudden physical strain, such as a cough, sneeze, or quick movement.

- Laboratory test results are an objective form of assessment data.

- Decreased renal function makes an elderly patient more susceptible to the development of renal calculi.

- Because elderly patients experience subcutaneous tissue redistribution and loss in areas such as the buttocks and deltoid muscles, the nurse should consider using shorter needles for injection of medication.

- Urge incontinence refers to the inability to suppress a sudden urge to urinate.

- Total incontinence is continuous urine leakage resulting from the bladder's inability to retain urine.

- Protein, vitamin, and mineral needs usually remain constant as a person ages, but caloric requirements decrease.

- Four valves keep blood flowing in one direction in the heart: two atrioventricular valves (tricuspid and mitral) and two semilunar valves (pulmonic and aortic).

- An elderly patient's height may decrease because of narrowing of the intervertebral spaces and exaggerated spinal curvature.

- The systems of measurement most often used in clinical practice are the metric system, apothecaries' system, and household system.

- Before signing an informed consent, a patient should understand what will occur during the preoperative, intraoperative, and postoperative phases; the risks involved; and the possible complications. The patient also should have a general idea of the time required from surgery to recovery and should have an opportunity to ask questions.

- A patient must sign a separate informed consent form for each procedure.

- Constipation most commonly occurs when the urge to defecate is suppressed and the muscles associated with bowel movements remain contracted.

- Gout develops in four stages: asymptomatic, acute, intercritical, and chronic.

- During percussion, the nurse uses quick, sharp tapping of the fingers or hands against body surfaces to produce sounds (that help determine the size, shape, position, and density of underlying organs and tissues), elicit tenderness, or assess reflexes.

- Ballottement is a form of light palpation involving gentle, repetitive bouncing of tissues against the hand and feeling their rebound.

- A foot cradle keeps bed linen off the patient's feet, which prevents skin irritation and breakdown, especially in a patient with peripheral vascular disease or neuropathy.

- If the patient is a married minor, permission to perform a procedure can be obtained from the patient's spouse.

- Gastric lavage is the flushing of the stomach and removal of ingested substances through a nasogastric tube. It can be used to treat poisoning or drug overdose.

- Common postoperative complications include hypovolemia, septicemia, septic shock, atelectasis, pneumonia, thrombophlebitis, and pulmonary embolism.

- An insulin pump delivers a continuous infusion of insulin into a selected subcutaneous site, commonly in the abdomen.

- During the evaluation step of the nursing process, the nurse assesses the patient's response to therapy.

- A common symptom of salicylate (aspirin) toxicity is tinnitus (ringing in the ears).

- Capillary refill time is the amount of time required for color to return to the nail bed after application of slight pressure, which causes blanching.

- Bruits are swishing sounds caused by turbulent blood flow. They commonly indicate a life- or limb-threatening vascular disease.

- A patient with Raynaud's disease should not smoke cigarettes or other tobacco products.

- O.U. means each eye; O.D., right eye; and O.S., left eye.

- Raynaud's disease is a primary arteriospastic disorder with no known cause; Raynaud's phenomenon, however, is caused by another disorder, such as scleroderma.

- To remove a foreign body from the eye, the nurse should irrigate the eye with sterile normal saline solution.

- When irrigating the eye, the nurse should direct the solution toward the lower conjunctival sac.

- Emergency care for a corneal injury from a caustic substance is eye flushing with copious amounts of water for 20 to 30 minutes.

- To remove a patient's artificial eye, the nurse depresses the lower lid.

- The nurse should use a soap-and-water solution to clean an artificial eye.

- Debridement is the mechanical, chemical, or surgical removal of necrotic tissue from a wound.

- Severe pain after cataract surgery indicates bleeding in the eye.

- The bivalve cast is cut into anterior and posterior portions to allow skin inspection.

• After ear irrigation, the nurse should place the patient on the affected side to permit gravity to drain fluid that remains in the ear.

• Ascites is an accumulation of fluid in the peritoneal cavity.

• A thready pulse is very fine and scarcely perceptible.

• If a patient with an indwelling (Foley) catheter reports abdominal discomfort, the nurse should assess for bladder distention, which may be caused by catheter blockage.

• Continuous bladder irrigation helps prevent urinary tract obstruction by flushing out small blood clots that form after prostate or bladder surgery.

• The nurse should remove an indwelling (Foley) catheter when bladder decompression is no longer needed, when the catheter is obstructed, or when the patient can resume voiding. (The longer a catheter remains in place, the greater the risk of urinary tract infection.)

• The extent of a burn injury can be determined by using the rule of nines: the head and neck are counted as 9%; each arm, as 9%; each leg, as 18%; the back of the trunk, as 18%; the front of the trunk, as 18%; and the perineum, as 1%.

• In a partial-thickness burn, the epidermis and dermis are affected.

• Axillary temperature usually is 1° F lower than oral temperature.

• After suctioning a tracheostomy tube, the nurse must document the color, amount, consistency, and odor of secretions.

• Nursing interventions for an asthma attack include administering oxygen and bronchodilators as prescribed, placing the patient in semi-Fowler's position, encouraging diaphragmatic breathing, and helping the patient relax.

- On a medication prescription, the abbreviation p.c. means that the medication should be administered after meals.

- After bladder irrigation, the nurse should document the amount, color, and clarity of the urine and the presence of clots or sediment.

- Prostate cancer usually is fatal if bone metastasis occurs.

- Laws regarding patient self-determination vary from state to state. Therefore, the nurse must be familiar with the laws of the state in which he or she works.

- *Gauge* refers to the inside diameter of a needle. The smaller the gauge, the larger the diameter.

- An adult normally has 32 permanent teeth.

- After turning a patient, the nurse should document the position used, time turned, and skin assessment findings.

- In a patient with increasing ICP, the level of responsiveness is the most significant indicator of the patient's condition.

- PERRLA is an abbreviation for normal pupil assessment findings: pupils equal, round, and reactive to light with accommodation.

- When percussing a patient's chest for postural drainage, the nurse's hands should be cupped.

- Regular insulin is the only insulin that can be mixed with other types of insulins.

- If a patient pulls out the outer tracheostomy tube, the nurse should hold open the tracheostomy with a surgical dilator until the physician provides appropriate care.

- When measuring a patient's pulse, the nurse should assess the rate, rhythm, quality, and strength.

• Before transferring a patient from a bed to a wheelchair, the nurse should push the wheelchair's footrests to the sides and lock its wheels.

• Tetralogy of Fallot consists of four defects: ventricular septal defect, overriding aorta, pulmonic stenosis, and right ventricular hypertrophy.

• When assessing respirations, the nurse should document the rate, rhythm, depth, and quality.

• For a subcutaneous injection, the nurse should use a ⅝", 25G needle.

• The medulla oblongata is the part of the brain that controls the respiratory center.

• For an unconscious patient, the nurse should perform passive range-of-motion exercises every 2 to 4 hours.

• Time-released medication is not recommended for use with a patient who has an ileostomy because it releases the drug at different rates along the GI tract.

• The notation "oriented times three" (or "O x 3") indicates that the patient is alert and oriented to person (knows who he or she is), place (knows where he or she is), and time (knows the date and time).

• Fluid intake includes all fluids taken by mouth, including foods that are liquid at room temperature, such as gelatin, custard, and ice cream. Fluid output includes urine, vomitus, and drainage (such as from a nasogastric tube or from a wound) as well as blood loss, diarrhea or stool, and perspiration.

• To perform an emergency cricothyrotomy, the nurse should make a small incision between the cricoid cartilage and the thyroid cartilage, insert a small tube into the opening and secure it, and attach the tube to an Ambu bag or other ventilation device.

• A patient's fluid intake usually is restricted for 24 hours before intravenous pyelography.

• After administering an intradermal injection, the nurse should not massage the area because massage can irritate the site and interfere with results.

• When administering an intradermal injection, the nurse should hold the syringe almost flat against the patient's skin (at about a 15-degree angle) with the bevel up.

• After a thyroidectomy, the patient should remain in semi-Fowler's position with the head firmly supported by pillows; neck flexion should be avoided.

• To obtain an accurate blood pressure, the nurse should inflate the manometer 20 to 30 mm Hg above the disappearance of the radial pulse before releasing the cuff pressure.

• A sodium polystyrene sulfonate (Kayexalate) enema, which exchanges sodium ions for potassium ions, is used to decrease the potassium level in a patient with hyperkalemia.

• If the color of a stoma is much lighter than when previously assessed, decreased circulation to the stoma may be present.

• Massage is contraindicated in a leg with a blood clot because it may dislodge the clot.

• The first place a nurse can detect jaundice is in the sclera of the eye.

• Jaundice is caused by excessive levels of conjugated or unconjugated bilirubin in the blood.

• Mydriatic drugs are used primarily to dilate the pupils for intraocular examinations.

• After eye surgery, the patient should be placed on the unaffected side.

• When assigning tasks to an LPN, the RN should delegate tasks that are considered bedside nursing care, such as taking vital signs, changing simple dressings, and giving baths.

• Deep calf pain on dorsiflexion of the foot is a positive Homans' sign, which suggests venous thrombosis or thrombophlebitis.

• Ultra short-acting barbiturates, such as thiopental sodium (Pentothal Sodium), are used as injection anesthetics in situations that require a short duration of anesthesia, such as outpatient surgery.

• Atropine sulfate may be used as a preanesthesia medication to reduce secretions and minimize vagal reflexes.

• The nursing care plan for a patient with infectious mononucleosis should emphasize strict bed rest during the acute febrile stage.

• During the acute phase of infectious mononucleosis, the patient should curtail activities to minimize the possibility of rupturing the enlarged spleen.

• Daily application of a long-acting, transdermal nitroglycerin patch is a convenient, effective way to prevent chronic angina. When applying such a patch, the nurse should avoid getting the medication on the hands.

• Tricyclic antidepressants are the drugs of choice for episodes of major depression.

• The nurse must wear a cap, gloves, gown, and mask when providing wound care to a burn patient.

• The nurse should expect to administer an analgesic before bathing a burn patient.

• The passage of black, tarry stools (melena) is a common sign of lower GI bleeding but also may occur in upper GI bleeding.

- The nurse should count an irregular pulse for 1 full minute.

- Spermatozoa (or their fragments) remain in the vagina for 72 hours after sexual intercourse.

- A patient with a gastric ulcer should avoid aspirin and aspirin-containing products because they can irritate the gastric mucosa.

- A patient who is vomiting while lying down should be placed in a lateral position to prevent aspiration of vomitus.

- A sitz bath (immersion of the pelvic area in tepid or hot water) usually takes 20 minutes.

- A low-fiber diet may contribute to the development of hemorrhoids.

- A patient with abdominal pain should not receive an analgesic until the cause of the pain is determined.

- If surgery requires hair removal, the Centers for Disease Control and Prevention recommend that a depilatory be used to avoid skin abrasions and cuts.

- For nasotracheal suctioning, the nurse should set wall suction at 50 to 95 mm Hg for an infant, 95 to 115 mm Hg for a child, or 80 to 120 mm Hg for an adult.

- The hallmark of tetralogy of Fallot is cyanosis, which usually appears several months after birth but may be present at birth if the infant has severe pulmonary stenosis.

- A change in pulse rate and rhythm may signal the onset of fatal arrhythmias in a patient who has had an MI.

- The best source of information for a patient's history usually is the patient.

- Prophylaxis is disease prevention.

• Palliative treatment relieves or reduces the intensity of uncomfortable symptoms but does not cure the causative disorder.

• Placing a postoperative patient in an upright position too quickly may produce hypotension.

• Body alignment is achieved when the body parts are in proper relation to their natural position.

• A high-carbohydrate, high-protein diet is the most therapeutic one for a postoperative patient.

• Trust is the foundation of a nurse-patient relationship.

• Blood pressure is the force exerted by the circulating volume of blood on arterial walls.

• Health care workers exposed to hepatitis B should receive hepatitis B immune globulin to prevent or modify symptoms of the disorder.

• A patient exposed to hepatitis B should receive 0.06 ml/kg I.M. of immune globulin within 72 hours after exposure and a repeat dose at 28 days after exposure.

• The nurse should advise a patient undergoing radiation therapy not to remove the markings on the skin made by the radiation therapist because these markings are landmarks for treatment.

• The most common symptom of osteoarthritis is joint pain—particularly after exercise or weight bearing—that usually is relieved by rest.

• *Malpractice* refers to a professional's wrongful conduct, improper discharge of duties, or failure to meet standards of care that cause harm to another.

• In adults, urine volume normally ranges from 800 to 2,000 ml/day and averages 1,200 to 1,500 ml/day.

- As a general rule, nurses cannot refuse a patient care assignment; however, they may refuse to participate in abortions in most states.

- *Negligence* refers to the failure to do something that reasonably could be expected to be done by a person in a given situation or the performance of an act that a reasonable and prudent person would not do.

- Directly applied moist heat softens crusts and exudates, penetrates deeper than dry heat, does not dry the skin, and usually is more comfortable for the patient.

- Tetracyclines seldom are considered drugs of choice for most common bacterial infections because their overuse has led to the emergence of tetracycline-resistant bacteria.

- Because light degrades nitroprusside sodium, the drug must be shielded from light. For example, an I.V. bag containing nitroprusside sodium must be wrapped in foil.

- Cephalosporins should be used cautiously in patients who are allergic to penicillin because such patients are more susceptible to hypersensitivity reactions.

- If chloramphenicol and penicillin must be administered concomitantly, the nurse should give the penicillin 1 or more hours before the chloramphenicol to avoid reduction in penicillin's bactericidal activity.

- The erythrocyte sedimentation rate measures the distance and speed that erythrocytes in whole blood have fallen in a vertical tube in 1 hour. The rate at which they fall to the bottom of the tube corresponds to the degree of inflammation.

- When teaching a patient with myasthenia gravis about pyridostigmine bromide (Mestinon) therapy, the nurse should stress the importance of taking the medication exactly as prescribed, on time, and in evenly spaced doses to prevent a relapse.

• If an antibiotic must be administered into a peripheral heparin lock, the nurse should flush the site with saline solution after the infusion to maintain I.V. patency.

• The nurse should instruct a patient with angina to take a nitroglycerin tablet before anticipated stress or exercise or, if the angina is nocturnal, at bedtime.

• ABG analysis evaluates gas exchange in the lungs (alveolar ventilation) by measuring the partial pressures of oxygen (PaO_2) and carbon dioxide ($PaCO_2$) and the pH of an arterial sample.

• The normal serum magnesium level ranges from 1.7 to 2.1 mg/dl or 1.5 to 2.5 mEq/liter.

• Patient preparation for a total cholesterol test includes an overnight fast and abstinence from alcohol for 24 hours before the test.

• The fasting plasma glucose test measures glucose levels after a 12- to 14-hour fast.

• The normal blood pH ranges from 7.35 to 7.45. A blood pH higher than 7.45 indicates alkalemia; one lower than 7.35 indicates acidemia.

• During the acid perfusion test, a small amount of weak hydrochloric acid solution is infused by way of a nasoesoph-ageal tube. A positive test result (pain after infusion) suggests reflux esophagitis.

• Normally, $PaCO_2$ ranges from 35 to 45 mm Hg. A $PaCO_2$ above 45 mm Hg indicates hypoventilation; one below 35 mm Hg indicates hyperventilation.

• Red cell indices aid in the diagnosis and classification of anemias.

• Normally, PaO_2 ranges from 80 to 100 mm Hg. A PaO_2 under 80 mm Hg indicates hypoxia.

- The WBC differential evaluates WBC distribution and morphology and provides more specific information about a patient's immune system than the WBC count.

- An exercise stress test (treadmill test, exercise ECG) continues until the patient reaches a predetermined target heart rate or experiences chest pain, fatigue, or other signs of exercise intolerance.

- Alterable risk factors for coronary artery disease include cigarette smoking, hypertension, high cholesterol or triglyceride levels, and diabetes.

- The mediastinum is the space between the lungs that contains the heart, esophagus, trachea, and other structures.

- Major complications of acute MI include arrhythmias, acute heart failure, cardiogenic shock, thromboembolism, and left ventricular rupture.

- The sinoatrial node is a cluster of hundreds of cells located in the right atrial wall near the opening of the superior vena cava.

- For one-person CPR, the ratio of compressions to ventilations is 15:2.

- For two-person CPR, the ratio of compressions to ventilations is 5:1.

- A patient with pulseless ventricular tachycardia is a candidate for defibrillation.

- Echocardiography, a noninvasive test that directs ultra–high-frequency sound waves through the chest wall into the heart, evaluates cardiac structure and function and can reveal valve deformities, tumors, septal defects, pericardial effusion, and idiopathic hypertrophic subaortic stenosis.

- *Ataxia* refers to an impaired ability to coordinate movements and results from a cerebellar or spinal cord lesion.

- On an ECG strip, each small block on the horizontal axis represents 0.04 seconds. Each large block (composed of five small blocks) represents 0.20 seconds.

- Starling's law states that the force of contraction of each heartbeat depends on the length of the muscle fibers of the heart wall.

- The therapeutic blood level for digoxin is 0.5 to 2.5 ng/ml.

- Pancrelipase (Pancrease) is used to treat steatorrhea, cystic fibrosis, and chronic pancreatitis.

- Treatment for mild-to-moderate varicose veins includes antiembolism stockings and an exercise program with walking to minimize venous pooling.

- According to Erikson, a young adult (ages 19 to 35) is in the developmental stage of intimacy versus isolation.

- States have enacted good Samaritan laws to encourage professionals to provide medical assistance at the scene of an accident without fear of a lawsuit arising from such assistance. These laws do not apply to care provided in a health care facility.

- A physician should sign verbal and telephone orders within the time period established by institutional policy, usually within 24 hours.

- A competent adult has the right to refuse lifesaving medical treatment; however, the individual should be fully informed of the consequences of this refusal.

- An intoxicated patient is not considered competent for the purposes of refusing required medical treatment and should not be allowed to check out of a hospital against medical advice.

- Florence Nightingale is considered the founder of modern nursing.

- Although a patient's health record or chart is the health care facility's physical property, its contents belong to the patient.

- Before a patient's record can be released to a third party, the patient or the patient's legal guardian must give written consent.

- Under the Controlled Substances Act, every dose of a controlled drug dispensed by the pharmacy must be accounted for, whether the dose was administered to a particular patient or discarded accidentally.

- A nurse cannot perform duties that violate a rule or regulation established by a state licensing board even if it is authorized by a health care facility or physician.

- The nurse should select a private room, preferably with a door that can be closed, to minimize interruptions during a patient interview.

- In categorizing nursing diagnoses, the nurse should address actual life-threatening problems first, followed by potentially life-threatening concerns.

- The major components of a nursing care plan are outcome criteria (patient goals) and nursing interventions.

- Standing orders, or protocols, establish guidelines for treating a particular disease or set of symptoms.

- Prolactin stimulates and sustains milk production.

- *Gynecomastia* refers to excessive mammary gland development and increased breast size in boys and men.

- The early stage of Alzheimer's disease lasts from 2 to 4 years and is manifested in inappropriate affect, transient paranoia, disorientation to time, memory loss, careless dressing, and impaired judgment.

• The middle stage of Alzheimer's disease lasts from 4 to 7 years and is marked by profound personality changes, loss of independence, disorientation, confusion, inability to recognize family members, and nocturnal restlessness.

• The last stage of Alzheimer's disease occurs during the final year of life and is manifested in a blank facial expression, seizures, loss of appetite, emaciation, irritability, and total dependence.

• Classic symptoms of Graves' disease are enlarged thyroid, nervousness, heat intolerance, weight loss despite increased appetite, sweating, diarrhea, tremor, and palpitations.

• Generalized malaise is a common symptom of viral and bacterial infections and depressive disorders.

• Vitamin C and protein are the most important nutrients in for wound healing.

• A patient with portal hypertension should receive vitamin K to promote active thrombin formation by the liver, which reduces the risk of bleeding.

• The nurse should administer a sedative cautiously to a patient with cirrhosis because the damaged liver cannot metabolize drugs effectively.

• Beta-hemolytic streptococcal infections should be treated, aggressively to prevent glomerulonephritis, rheumatic fever, and other complications.

• The most common nosocomial infection is urinary tract infection.

• The nurse should implement strict isolation precautions to protect a patient with a burn infected by *Staphylococcus aureus*.

• A patient undergoing external radiation therapy should not apply cream or lotion to the treatment site.

- Strabismus is a normal finding in a neonate.

- The most common vascular complication of diabetes mellitus is atherosclerosis.

- Insulin deficiency may result in hyperglycemia.

- Signs of Parkinson's disease include drooling, mask-like expression, and propulsive gait.

- I.V. cholangiography is contraindicated in a patient with hyperthyroidism, severe renal or hepatic damage, tuberculosis, or iodine hypersensitivity.

- In assessing a patient's heart, the nurse normally finds the point of maximal impulse at the 5th intercostal space near the apex.

- The S_1 sound heard on auscultation is caused by closure of the mitral and tricuspid valves.

- Threatening a patient with an injection for failing to take an oral medication is an example of assault.

- The coronary artery supplies blood to the myocardium.

- A patient with gouty arthritis should increase the fluid intake to prevent calculi formation.

- Anxiety is the most common cause of chest pain.

- A patient on a low-salt diet should avoid canned vegetables.

- Bananas are a good source of potassium and should be included in a low-salt diet for a patient taking a potassium-wasting diuretic, such as furosemide (Lasix).

- The nurse should encourage a patient at risk of pneumonia to turn frequently, cough, and breathe deeply. These actions mobilize pulmonary secretions, promote alveolar gas exchange, and help prevent atelectasis.

- The nurse should notify the physician any time a patient's blood pressure reaches 180/100 mm Hg.

- Buck's traction is used to immobilize and reduce spasms in a fractured hip.

- For a patient with a fractured hip, the nurse should assess neurocirculatory status every 2 hours.

- When caring for a patient with a fractured hip, the nurse should use pillows or trochanter rolls to maintain abduction.

- Orthopnea is a symptom of left ventricular failure.

- Although a fiberglass cast is more durable and dries faster than a plaster cast, it frequently causes skin irritation.

- The major circulatory complication of an immobilized patient is pulmonary embolism.

- To relieve edema in a fractured limb, the patient should keep the limb elevated.

- I.V. antibiotics are the treatment of choice for a patient with osteomyelitis.

- A postpartal patient may resume sexual intercourse when perineal and uterine wounds have healed (usually within 4 weeks after delivery).

- Blue dye in cimetidine (Tagamet) can cause a false-positive result on a fecal occult blood test, such as a Hemoccult test.

- A pregnant staff member should not be assigned to work with a patient who has a cytomegalovirus infection.

- The nurse should suspect elder abuse if wounds are inconsistent with the history, multiple wounds are present, or wounds are in different stages of healing.

- *Fetal demise* refers to death of the fetus after viability.

- Immediately after amputation, patient care includes monitoring drainage from the stump, positioning the affected arm or leg, assisting with exercises prescribed by a physical therapist, and wrapping and conditioning the stump.

- Premature infants develop respiratory distress syndrome because their alveoli lack surfactant.

- A patient who is prone to constipation should increase the bulk intake by eating whole-grain cereals and fresh fruits and vegetables.

- The most common method of inducing labor after artificial rupture of the membrane is oxytocin (Pitocin) infusion.

- The speculum used in the pelvic examination of a rape victim should be lubricated with water because commercial lubricants retard sperm motility and interfere with specimen collection and analysis.

- Physical comfort is the top priority in nursing care for a terminally ill patient.

- Dorsiflexion of the foot provides immediate relief of leg cramps.

- After cardiac surgery, the patient should limit daily sodium intake to 2 g and daily cholesterol intake to 300 mg.

- After the patient's amniotic membranes rupture, the priority nursing action is monitoring the FHR.

- Bleeding after intercourse is an early sign of cervical cancer.

- Oral hypoglycemic agents stimulate insulin release from beta cells in the islets of Langerhans of the pancreas.

- When visiting a patient with a radiation implant, family members and friends must limit their stay to 10 minutes.

- Common causes of vaginal infection include using an antibiotic, oral contraceptive, or corticosteroid; wearing tight-fitting panty hose; and having sexual intercourse with an infected partner.

- A patient with a radiation implant should be maintained in isolation until the implant is removed. The nurse should carefully plan the time spent with the patient to minimize radiation exposure, which increases with time.

- Among cultural groups, native Americans have the lowest incidence of cancer.

- The kidneys filter blood, selectively reabsorb substances needed to maintain the constancy of body fluid, and excrete metabolic wastes.

- Re-examination of life goals is a major developmental task during middle adulthood.

- To prevent straining during defecation, docusate sodium (Colace) is the laxative of choice for patients recovering from MI, rectal surgery, or postpartal constipation.

- Delirium tremens, or DTs (an acute psychotic reaction triggered by alcohol withdrawal), begin with anorexia, insomnia, headache, and restlessness and escalate to a syndrome that includes agitation, disorientation, vivid hallucinations, and tremors of the hands, feet, legs, and tongue.

- In a hospitalized alcoholic, DTs most commonly occur 3 to 4 days after admission.

- Confrontation is a communication technique in which the nurse points out discrepancies between the patient's words and nonverbal behaviors.

- Telangiectatic nevi (stork bites) are normal neonatal skin lesions characterized by flat red or purple areas on the back of the neck, upper eyelids, upper lip, and bridge of the nose. They regress by age 2.

• After prostate surgery, a patient's primary sources of pain are bladder spasms and irritation in the area around the catheter.

• Toxoplasmosis is more likely to affect a pregnant cat owner than other pregnant women because cat feces in the litter box harbor the infecting organism.

• The most common reasons for cesarean birth are malpresentation, fetal distress, cephalopelvic disproportion, certain cases of toxemia, previous cesarean birth, and inadequate progress in labor.

• The nurse should suspect placenta previa in a pregnant patient with painless bleeding and should prepare her for ultrasonography.

• Amniocentesis increases the risk of spontaneous abortion, trauma to the fetus or placenta, premature labor, infection, and Rh sensitization of the fetus.

• After amniocentesis, abdominal cramping or spontaneous vaginal bleeding may indicate complications.

• An Rh-negative primigravida should receive $Rh_o(D)$ immune globulin (RhoGAM) after delivering an Rh-positive infant to prevent her from developing Rh antibodies.

• If a pregnant patient's test results are negative for glucose but positive for acetone, the nurse should assess the patient's diet for inadequate caloric intake.

• Calcium deficiency and lack of proper exercise can result in leg cramps during pregnancy.

• Good food sources of folic acid include leafy green vegetables, liver, and legumes.

• Rubella infection in a pregnant patient, especially during the first trimester, can lead to spontaneous abortion or stillbirth as well as fetal cardiac and other birth defects.

- The Glasgow Coma Scale evaluates verbal, eye, and motor responses to determine level of consciousness (LOC).

- To calculate fluid replacement for a burn patient, the nurse should use the following formula: 2 ml x body weight (in kilograms) x the percentage of the burned surface area. This formula yields the amount of fluid to be administered in the first 24 hours. Half the amount should be given in the first 8 hours; the other half, in the next 16 hours.

- The nurse should place an unconscious patient in low Fowler's position for intermittent nasogastric tube feedings.

- Laennec's (alcoholic) cirrhosis is the most common type of cirrhosis.

- In decorticate posturing, the patient's arms are adducted and flexed, with the wrists and fingers flexed on the chest. The legs are stiffly extended and internally rotated, with plantar flexion of the feet.

- For a patient with drug-induced psychosis, the time of drug ingestion can help determine if the drug can be evacuated from the body.

- A pregnant patient may receive a prescription for an iron supplement to help prevent anemia.

- Direct antiglobulin (direct Coombs') test is used to detect maternal antibodies attached to RBCs in the neonate.

- The most common intra-abdominal tumor in children is Wilms' tumor (nephroblastoma).

- A patient who is a potential candidate for surgery should receive nothing by mouth (NPO) from 12:00 midnight of the day before surgery until cleared by a physician.

- Nausea and vomiting during the first trimester of pregnancy are caused by rising levels of the hormone human chorionic gonadotropin (hCG).

- In an infant, feeding problems, such as fatigue, tachypnea, and irritability during feeding, may be early signs of a congenital heart defect.

- Meperidine (Demerol) is an effective analgesic for relieving the pain of nephrolithiasis (urinary calculi)

- An injured patient with thrombocytopenia is at risk of life-threatening internal and external hemorrhage.

- The Trendelenburg gait test is used to check for unilateral hip dislocation.

- As soon as possible after death, the patient should be placed in the supine position with the arms at the sides and the head on a pillow.

- Vascular resistance depends on blood viscosity, vessel length, and, most important, inside vessel diameter.

- A below-the-knee amputation leaves the knee intact for prosthesis application and allows a more normal gait.

- Cerebrospinal fluid (CSF) flows through and protects the four ventricles of the brain, the subarachnoid space, and the spinal canal.

- Sodium regulates extracellular osmolality.

- The heart and brain can maintain blood circulation in the early stages of shock.

- After limb amputation, narcotic analgesics may not relieve "phantom limb" pain.

- A patient who receives multiple blood transfusions is at risk of developing hypocalcemia.

- Syphilis initially causes painless chancres (small, fluid-filled lesions) on the genitals and sometimes on other parts of the body.

- Exposure to a radioactive source is controlled by time (limiting time spent with patient), distance (from the patient), and shielding (type used).

- Jaundice is a sign of dysfunction, not a disease.

- Severe jaundice can result in brain stem dysfunction if the unconjugated bilirubin level in blood is elevated to 20 to 25 mg/dl.

- The patient should take cimetidine (Tagamet) with meals to help ensure a consistent therapeutic effect.

- When caring for a patient with jaundice, the nurse should relieve pruritus by providing a soothing lotion or baking soda bath and should prevent bleeding by keeping the patient's fingernails short.

- Type B hepatitis, which is generally transmitted parenterally, also can be spread through contact with human secretions and feces.

- Insulin is a naturally occurring hormone secreted by the beta cells of the islets of Langerhans in the pancreas in response to a rise in the blood glucose level.

- Diabetes mellitus is a chronic endocrine disorder characterized by insulin deficiency or resistance to insulin by body tissues.

- A diagnosis of diabetes mellitus is based on the classic symptoms (polyuria, polyphagia, weight loss, and polydipsia) and a random blood glucose level above 200 mg/dl or a fasting plasma glucose level above 140 mg/dl on two testings.

- A patient with non-insulin-dependent (Type II) diabetes mellitus produces some insulin and does not need exogenous insulin supplementation under normal circumstances. Most patients with this type of diabetes respond well to oral hypoglycemics, which stimulate the pancreas to increase insulin synthesis and release.

- A patient with insulin-dependent (Type I) diabetes mellitus cannot produce endogenous insulin and requires exogenous insulin administration to meet the body's needs.

- Rapid-acting insulins are clear; intermediate- and long-acting insulins are turbid (cloudy).

- Rapid-acting insulins begin to act in 30 to 60 minutes, reach a peak concentration in 2 to 10 hours, and have a duration of action of 5 to 16 hours.

- Blood glucose normally ranges from 65 to 130 mg/dl.

- The best times to test the patient's glucose level are before each meal and at bedtime.

- Intermediate-acting insulins begin to act in 1 to 2 hours, reach a peak concentration in 4 to 15 hours, and have a duration of action of 22 to 28 hours.

- Long-acting insulins begin to act in 4 to 8 hours, reach a peak concentration in 10 to 30 hours, and have a duration of action of 36 or more hours.

- A patient with above-normal glucose levels after glucose administration in a nonfasting glucose test but with normal plasma glucose levels otherwise has impaired glucose tolerance.

- Insulin requirements are increased by growth, pregnancy, increased food intake, stress, surgery, infection, illness, increased insulin antibodies, and some medications.

- Insulin requirements are decreased by hypothyroidism, decreased food intake, exercise, and some medications.

- Hypoglycemia occurs when the blood glucose level falls below 50 mg/dl.

- An insulin-resistant patient is one who requires more than 200 units of insulin each day.

- Hypoglycemia may occur 1 to 3 hours after administration of a rapid-acting insulin; 4 to 18 hours after administration of an intermediate-acting insulin; and 18 to 30 hours after administration of a long-acting insulin.

- When the blood glucose level falls rapidly, the patient may experience sweating, tremors, pallor, tachycardia, and palpitations.

- Objective signs of hypoglycemia include slurred speech, lack of coordination, staggered gait, seizures, and, possibly, coma.

- A conscious patient with hypoglycemia should receive sugar in a form that can be swallowed, such as orange juice, candy, or lump sugar.

- An unconscious patient with hypoglycemia should receive a subcutaneous or an I.M. injection of glucagon as prescribed by a physician.

- A patient with diabetes mellitus should inspect the feet daily for calluses, corns, or blisters; wash the feet with warm water; and trim the toenails straight across to prevent ingrown toenails.

- The early stage of ketoacidosis is manifested by polyuria, polydipsia, anorexia, muscle cramps, and vomiting; the late stage, by Kussmaul's respirations, sweet breath odor, and stupor or coma.

- An allergen is a substance capable of producing a hypersensitivity reaction.

- To maintain package sterility, the nurse should open the wrapper's top flap away from the body, open each side flap by touching only the outer part of the wrapper, and open the final flap by grasping the turned-down corner and pulling it toward the body.

- A corrective lens for nearsightedness is concave.

• Chronic untreated hypothyroidism or abrupt withdrawal of thyroid medication may lead to myxedema coma.

• Signs and symptoms of myxedema coma are lethargy, stupor, decreased LOC, dry skin and hair, delayed deep tendon reflexes, progressive respiratory center depression and cerebral hypoxia, weight gain, hypothermia, and hypoglycemia.

• Nearsightedness occurs when the focal point of a ray of light from an object that is 20 ft (6 m) away falls in front of the retina.

• Farsightedness occurs when the focal point of a ray of light from an object that is 20 ft (6 m) away falls behind the retina.

• A corrective lens for farsightedness is convex.

• *Refraction* refers to clinical measurement of the error in eye focusing.

• Adhesions are bands of granulation and scar tissue that develop in some patients after a surgical incision.

• The nurse should moisten an eye patch for an unconcious patient because a dry patch may irritate the cornea.

• A patient who has had eye surgery should not bend over, comb the hair vigorously, or engage in activity that increases intraocular pressure.

• When caring for a patient with a penetrating eye injury, the nurse should loosely patch both eyes with sterile gauze, administer an oral antibiotic (in high doses) and tetanus injection as prescribed, and refer the patient to an ophthalmologist for follow-up.

• Signs and symptoms of colorectal cancer include changes in bowel habits, rectal bleeding, abdominal pain, anorexia, weight loss, malaise, anemia, and constipation or diarrhea.

• When climbing stairs with crutches, the patient should lead with the uninvolved leg and follow with the crutches and involved leg.

• When descending stairs with crutches, the patient should lead with the crutches and the involved leg and follow with the uninvolved leg.

• When surgery requires eyelash trimming, the nurse should apply petrolatum jelly to the scissor blades so that the eyelashes will adhere to them.

• Pain after a corneal transplant may indicate that the dressing has been applied too tightly, the graft has slipped, or the eye is hemorrhaging.

• A patient with retinal detachment may report floating spots, flashes of light, and a sensation of a veil or curtain coming down.

• Preoperative care for a patient with retinal detachment includes bandaging both eyes and restricting activities until the anesthetic has worn off.

• Postoperative care for a patient with retinal detachment includes avoiding bumping the patient's head or bed, encouraging deep breathing but not coughing, and instructing the patient to avoid hand work and walking until approved by the physician.

• A patient with a cataract may report vision disturbances, such as image distortion, light glaring, and gradual vision loss.

• When talking to a hearing impaired patient who can lip read, the nurse should speak slowly and enunciate clearly, point to objects as needed, avoid chewing gum, and face the patient.

• Meniere's disease is manifested in this triad of symptoms: severe vertigo, hearing loss, and tinnitus.

- The fluorescent treponemal antibody absorption (FTA-ABS) test is a specific serologic test for syphilis.

- The nurse may use a sponge bath with tepid water (80° to 93° F [26° to 34° C]) to reduce fever.

- When communicating with a patient who has had a CVA, the nurse should allow ample time for the patient to speak and respond, face the patient's unaffected side, avoid talking fast, give visual clues, supplement speech with gestures, and give instructions consistently.

- The major complication of Bell's palsy is keratitis (corneal inflammation), which results from incomplete eye closure on the affected side.

- Immunosuppressants are used to combat tissue rejection and help control autoimmune disorders.

- After a unilateral CVA, a patient may be able to propel a wheelchair by using a heel-to-toe movement with the unaffected leg and turning the wheel with the unaffected hand.

- First morning urine is the most concentrated and most likely to reveal abnormalities. It should be refrigerated to retard bacterial growth or, for microscopic examination, should be sent to the laboratory immediately.

- The patient recovering from a CVA should align the arms and legs correctly, wear high-top sneakers to prevent footdrop and contracture, and use an egg crate, flotation, or pulsating mattress to help prevent pressure ulcers.

- After an arm or leg fracture, the bone may display complete union (normal healing), delayed union (healing that takes longer than expected), or nonunion (failure to heal).

- The most common complication of a hip fracture is thromboembolism, which may occlude an artery and cause the area it supplies to become cold and cyanotic.

- Chloral hydrate suppositories should be refrigerated.

- Cast application usually requires two persons; it should not be attempted alone.

- A plaster cast reaches maximum strength in 48 hours; a synthetic cast, within 30 minutes because it does not require drying.

- Severe pain indicates pressure ulcer development within a cast; the pain decreases significantly once an ulcer develops.

- With running traction (Buck's traction), the patient may not be turned without disrupting the line of pull; with balanced suspension traction, the patient may be elevated, turned slightly, and moved as needed.

- Indications of circulatory interference are abnormal skin coolness, cyanosis, and rubor or pallor.

- During the postoperative phase, a rising pulse rate and falling blood pressure may indicate hemorrhage and impending shock.

- Orthopedic surgical wounds bleed more than other surgical wounds. The nurse can expect 200 to 500 ml of drainage during the first 24 hours and less than 30 ml each 8 hours for the next 48 hours.

- A patient who has had hip surgery should not adduct or flex the operated hip because flexion greater than 90 degrees may cause dislocation.

- The Hoyer lift, a hydraulic device, enables two persons to lift and move a nonambulatory patient safely.

- A patient with carpal tunnel syndrome, a complex of symptoms caused by median nerve compression in the carpal tunnel, usually reports weakness, pain, burning, numbness, or tingling in one or both hands.

- The nurse should not use a cotton-tipped applicator to dry a patient's ear canal or remove wax because it may force cerumen against the tympanic membrane.

- The nurse should remove a patient's ice bag for 30 minutes at least every 2 hours to prevent maceration and tissue ischemia from diminished blood flow to the area.

- A patient's identification bracelet should remain in place until the patient has been discharged from the health care facility and has left the building.

- The nurse should instruct a patient who has had heat-stroke to wear light-colored loose-fitting clothing, rest frequently, and drink plenty of fluids.

- A conscious patient with heat exhaustion or heatstroke should receive a solution of ½ teaspoon of salt in 120 ml of water every 15 minutes for 1 hour.

- An I.V. line inserted during an emergency or outside the hospital setting should be changed within 24 hours.

- The nurse should discontinue the tepid bath and notify the physician if the patient develops cyanosis or a change in pulse rate or respirations.

- After a tepid bath, the nurse should dry the patient thoroughly to prevent chills.

- The nurse should take the patient's temperature 30 minutes after completing a tepid bath.

- Shower or bath water should not exceed 105° F (40.5° C).

- Dilatation and curettage (D&C) is the widening of the cervical canal with a dilator and the scraping of the uterus with a curette.

- When not in use, all central venous catheters must be capped with p.r.n. adaptors after flushing.

- Care after a D&C consists of bed rest for 1 day, mild analgesics for pain, and use of a sterile pad for as long as bleeding persists.

- If a patient feels faint during a bath or shower, the nurse should turn off the water, cover the patient, lower the patient's head, and summon help.

- For the first few months of levothyroxine sodium (Synthroid) therapy, a child may experience temporary hair loss.

- A patient taking oral contraceptives should not smoke because smoking can intensify the drug's adverse cardiovascular effects.

- The use of soft restraints, such as a Posey safety vest, requires a physician's order as well as assessment and documentation of the patient and affected limbs, according to facility policy.

- A vest restraint should be used cautiously in a patient with CHF or a respiratory disorder because it can tighten with movement, further limiting respiratory function. Also, the least amount of restraint should be used to ensure patient safety.

- If a piggyback system becomes dislodged, the nurse should replace the entire piggyback system with the appropriate solution and medication as prescribed.

- The nurse should not secure a restraint to the bed's side rails because they might be inadvertently lowered, causing patient injury or discomfort.

- Before discharging a patient who has had an abortion, the nurse should instruct her to report bright red clots, bleeding that lasts longer than 7 days, or signs of infection, such as a temperature above 100° F (37.8° C), foul-smelling vaginal discharge, severe uterine cramping, nausea, or vomiting.

• The nurse should assess a patient with limb restraints every 2 hours to detect signs of impaired circulation.

• The CDCP recommends using a needleless system for piggybacking an I.V. medication into the main I.V. line.

• Handwashing is essential upon entering and leaving the room of a patient in isolation because the hands are considered contaminated.

• If a mask is required, it should cover the mouth and nose and should not be reused after removal.

• If a gown is required, the nurse should put it on upon entering the patient's room and discard it upon leaving.

• When changing the dressing of a patient in isolation, the nurse should wear two pairs of gloves.

• The duration of pregnancy averages 280 days, 40 weeks, 9 calendar months, or 10 lunar months.

• A disposable bedpan and urinal should remain in the room of a patient in isolation and be discarded on discharge or at the end of the isolation period.

• Mycoses (fungal infections) may be systemic or deep (affecting the internal organs), subcutaneous (involving the skin), or superficial (growing on the outer layer of skin and hair).

• The night before a sputum specimen is to be collected by expectoration, the patient should increase fluid intake to promote sputum production.

• A stool sample for an ova and parasite study should be collected directly into a waterproof container, covered with a lid, and sent immediately to the laboratory. If the patient is bedridden, the sample can be collected into a clean, dry bedpan and then transferred with a tongue depressor into a container.

- When obtaining a sputum specimen for testing, the nurse should instruct the patient to rinse the mouth with clean water, cough deeply from the chest, and expectorate into a sterile container.

- Tonometry allows indirect measurement of intraocular pressure and aids in early detection of glaucoma.

- Pulmonary function tests (a series of measurements that evaluate ventilatory function through spirometric measurements) help diagnose pulmonary dysfunction.

- After a liver biopsy, the patient should lay on the right side to compress the biopsy site, which decreases the possibility of bleeding.

- A patient with cirrhosis should follow a diet that restricts sodium but provides protein, vitamins (especially B, C, and K and folate), and at least 3,000 calories a day.

- If 12 hours of suction therapy do not relieve bowel obstruction, surgery is indicated.

- The nurse can puncture a nifedipine (Procardia) capsule with a needle, withdraw its liquid, and instill it into the buccal pouch.

- When administering whole blood or packed RBCs, the nurse should use a 16G or 18G needle or cannula to avoid RBC hemolysis.

- Hirsutism is excessive body hair in a masculine distribution.

- The Controlled Substances Act designated five categories, or schedules, that classify controlled drugs according to their abuse liability.

- Schedule I drugs, such as heroin, have a high abuse potential and have no currently accepted medical use in the United States.

- Schedule II drugs, such as morphine, opium, and meperidine, have a high abuse potential but have currently accepted medical uses. Their use may lead to physical or psychological dependence.

- Schedule III drugs, such as paregoric and butabarbital, have a lower abuse potential than Schedule I or II drugs. Abuse of Schedule III drugs may lead to moderate or low physical or psychological dependence, or both.

- Schedule IV drugs, such as chloral hydrate, have a low abuse potential compared with Schedule III drugs.

- Schedule V drugs, such as cough syrups that contain codeine, have the lowest abuse potential of the controlled substances.

- One unit of whole blood or packed RBCs should be administered over 2 to 4 hours.

- For I.V. medication administration in an infant or an older patient with small veins, the nurse should use a 21G or 23G winged set, dilute the medication as prescribed, and infuse it slowly to prevent vein injury.

- A $PaCO_2$ level below 35 mm Hg suggests respiratory alkalosis.

- A vitamin is an organic compound that usually cannot be synthesized by the body and is needed in metabolic processes.

- An adolescent's eating habits are significantly influenced by the peer group.

- In an infant, manifestations of hypothyroidism are inactivity, excessive sleeping, and minimal crying.

- Pulmonary embolism can be caused by thromboembolism of fat, blood, bone marrow, or amniotic fluid obstructing the pulmonary artery.

- After maxillofacial surgery, a patient whose mandible and maxilla have been wired together should keep a pair of scissors or wire cutters readily available to prevent aspiration if vomiting occurs.

- Rapid instillation of fluid during colonic irrigation can cause abdominal cramping.

- A collaborative environment between health care workers helps shorten the hospital stay and increase patient satisfaction.

- Predictable hazards for elderly patients in a health care facility include nighttime confusion (sundowning), fractures from falling, immobility-induced pressure ulcers, prolonged convalescence, and loss of home and support systems.

- Respiratory tract infections—especially viral ones—can trigger asthma attacks.

- Oxygen therapy is used in severe asthma attacks to prevent or treat hypoxemia.

- During an asthma attack, the patient may prefer nasal prongs to a Venturi mask because of the mask's smothering effect.

- COPD usually develops over a period of years and results from smoking in 95% of patients.

- An early sign of COPD is slowing of forced expiration. A healthy person can empty the lungs in less than 4 seconds; a patient with COPD may take 6 to 10 seconds.

- COPD eventually leads to structural changes in the lungs, including overdistended alveoli and hyperinflated lungs.

- Cystic fibrosis, which is transmitted as an autosomal recessive trait, causes dysfunction of the exocrine gland, sweat glands, and resiratory and digestive systems.

• A common manifestation of cystic fibrosis in infancy is meconium ileus caused by obstruction of the small intestine by viscous meconium.

• Infants who have cystic fibrosis but do not have meconium ileus at birth have good appetites but gain weight slowly.

• Cellulitis is manifested as localized heat, redness, swelling, and, occasionally, fever, chills, and malaise.

• The initial weight loss for a healthy neonate is 5% to 10% of the birth weight.

• The hemoglobin value in neonates normally ranges from 17 to 20 g/dl.

• Venous stasis may precipitate thrombophlebitis.

• Thrombophlebitis treatment includes leg elevation, heat application, and, possibly, anticoagulant therapy.

• A suctioning machine should remain at the bedside of a patient who has had maxillofacial surgery.

• The nurse may use the PLISSIT model for intervening with patients who have sexual problems. The acronym stands for giving Permission, providing Limited Information, making Specific Suggestions, and referring for Intensive Therapy.

• *Crowning* describes the appearance of the fetus's head when its largest diameter is encircled by the vulvovaginal ring.

• If an immunization schedule is interrupted for any reason, it should be restarted from the last immunization administered and not from the beginning.

• In passive range-of-motion exercises, the therapist moves the patient's joints through as full a range of motion as possible to improve or maintain joint mobility and help prevent contractures.

- In resistance exercises, which allow muscle length to change, the patient performs exercises against resistance applied by the therapist.

- In isometric exercises, the patient contracts muscles against stable resistance but without joint movement. The muscle length remains the same, but muscle strength and tone may increase.

- Predisposing factors for impetigo (a contagious, superficial, vesicopustular skin infection) include poor hygiene, anemia, malnutrition, and a warm climate.

- Activities of daily living are actions that the patient must perform every day to provide self-care and interact with society.

- Once CPR begins, it should not be interrupted, except when a rescuer is alone and must summon help. In such a case, the rescuer should perform CPR for 1 minute before calling for help.

- The tongue is the most common airway obstruction in an unconscious patient.

- For adult CPR, the chest compression rate is 80 to 100 times per minute.

- A patient with ulcers should avoid bedtime snacks because food may stimulate nocturnal secretions.

- In angioplasty, a blood vessel is dilated by a balloon catheter inserted through the skin and the vessel's lumen to the narrowed area. Once in place, the balloon is inflated to flatten plaque against the vessel wall.

- A full liquid diet supplies nutrients, fluids, and calories in simple, easily digested foods, such as apple juice, cream of wheat, milk, coffee, strained cream soup, high-protein gelatin, cranberry juice, custard, and ice cream. It is prescribed for patients who cannot tolerate a regular diet.

• A pureed diet meets the patient's nutritional needs without foods that are difficult for the patient to chew or swallow.

• A soft, or light, diet is specifically designed for patients who have difficulty chewing or tolerating a regular diet. It is nutritionally adequate and consists of such foods as orange juice, cream of wheat, scrambled eggs, enriched toast, cream of chicken soup, wheat bread, fruit cocktail, and mushroom soup.

• A regular diet is provided for patients who do not require diet modification.

• A pediatric diet normally is ordered as "diet for age" by the physician. It should include sufficient nutrients and calories to promote growth and development.

• A bland diet restricts foods that cause gastric irritation or produce acid secretion without providing a neutralizing effect.

• A clear liquid diet provides fluid and a gradual return to a regular diet; however, it is deficient in all nutrients and the patient should consume this diet for only a short period.

• Patients with a gastric ulcer should avoid alcohol, caffeinated beverages, aspirin, and spicy foods.

• In active assistance exercises, the patient performs exercises with the therapist's help.

• Penicillinase is an enzyme produced by certain bacteria. It converts penicillin into an inactive product, thereby increasing the bacteria's resistance to the antibiotic.

• Battle's sign is a bluish discoloration behind the ear in some patients who sustain a basilar skull fracture.

• Crackles are nonmusical clicking or rattling noises heard during auscultation of abnormal breath sounds. They result from air passing through fluid-filled airways.

• Antibiotics are not effective against viruses, protozoa, or parasites.

• Most penicillins and cephalosporins produce their antibiotic effects by cell wall inhibition.

• When assessing a patient with an inguinal hernia, the nurse should suspect strangulation if the patient reports severe pain, nausea, and vomiting.

• Phimosis is tightness of the prepuce of the penis that prevents foreskin retraction over the glans.

• Aminoglycosides are natural antibiotics that are effective against gram-negative bacteria. They must be used with caution because they can cause nephrotoxicity and ototoxicity.

• Upon scrotal examination, varicoceles and tumors do not transilluminate, but spermatoceles and hydroceles do.

• The heart of a child with tetralogy of Fallot appears boot-shaped on X-ray films because the right ventricle is enlarged.

• Testing of the six cardinal fields of gaze evaluates the function of all extraocular muscles and cranial nerves III, IV, and VI.

• A hordeoleum (eyelid stye) represents an infection of one or more sebaceous glands of the eyelid.

• A chalazion is an eyelid mass that results from chronic inflammation of the meibomian gland.

• During an ophthalmoscopic examination, the absence of the red reflex indicates a lens opacity (cataract) or a detached retina.

• Respiratory acidosis is associated with such conditions as drug overdose, Guillain-Barré syndrome, myasthenia gravis, COPD, pickwickian syndrome, and kyphoscoliosis.

• Respiratory alkalosis is associated with such conditions as high fever, severe hypoxia, asthma, and pulmonary embolism.

• Metabolic acidosis is associated with such conditions as renal failure, diarrhea, diabetic ketosis, and lactic ketosis and with high doses of acetazolamide (Diamox).

• Gastrectomy is the surgical excision of all or part of the stomach to remove a chronic peptic ulcer, to stop hemorrhage in the perforated ulcer, or to remove a malignant tumor.

• Metabolic alkalosis is associated with nasal and gastric suctioning, excessive diuretic use, and steroid therapy.

• Vitiligo (a benign, acquired skin disease) is marked by stark-white skin patches resulting from the destruction and loss of pigment cells.

• A multipara is a woman who has has two or more pregnancies that progressed to viability (whether or not the offspring were alive at birth).

• Overdose or accidental overingestion of disulfiram (Antabuse) should be treated by gastric aspiration or lavage along with supportive therapy.

• The six types of heart murmurs are graded from I to VI. A grade VI heart murmur can be heard with the stethoscope slightly raised from the chest.

• The causes of abdominal distention are represented by the six Fs: flatus, feces, fetus, fluid, fat, and fatal (malignant) neoplasm.

• A positive Murphy's sign indicates cholecystitis.

• Signs of appendicitis include right abdominal pain, abdominal rigidity and rebound tenderness, nausea, and anorexia.

• Ascites can be detected when more than 500 ml of fluid has collected in the intraperitoneal space.

• The most important goal to include in a care plan is the patient's goal.

• The ideal environment for a patient with organic brain syndrome or a senile disease is one that is stable and limits confusion.

• Memory loss in organic brain syndrome usually affects all spheres but begins with recent memory loss.

• In a pregnant patient, preeclampsia may progress to eclampsia, which is characterized by seizures and may lead to coma.

• The nurse assigns an Apgar score to a neonate at 1 and 5 minutes after birth. The score is based on respiratory effort, heart rate, muscle tone, reflex irritability, and color.

• During cardiac catheterization, the patient may experience a thudding sensation in the chest, a strong desire to cough, and a transient feeling of heat, usually in the head, from the contrast medium injection.

• Insulin requirements increase during the third trimester because of the anti-insulin effects of placental hormones.

• Gestational age can be estimated by ultrasound measurement of abdominal circumference, femur length, and fetal head size. Such measurements are most accurate between 12 and 18 weeks' gestation.

• Skeletal system abnormalities and ventricular septal defects are the most common disorders of infants born to diabetic women. The incidence of congenital malformation is three times higher in these infants than in those born to nondiabetic women.

- Slight bubbling in the suction column of a thoracic drainage system, such as a Pleur-evac unit, indicates that it is working properly; a lack of bubbling in the suction chamber indicates inadequate suction.

- Nutritional deficiency is a common finding in people who have a long history of alcohol abuse.

- Treatment for alcohol withdrawal may include administration of I.V. glucose for hypoglycemia, I.V. fluid containing thiamine and other B vitamins, and antianxiety, antidiarrheal, anticonvulsant, and antiemetic drugs.

- An alcoholic patient receives thiamine to help prevent peripheral neuropathy and Korsakoff's syndrome.

- Because alcohol lowers the seizure threshold in some people, alcohol withdrawal may precipitate seizure activity.

- Paraphrasing is an active listening technique in which the nurse restates what a patient has just conveyed.

- A patient with Korsakoff's syndrome may use confabulation to cover memory lapses or periods of amnesia.

- The most common symptom of type A hepatitis is anorexia. Other early effects include chills, nausea, vomiting, dyspepsia, and liver tenderness.

- Nonviral hepatitis usually results from exposure to certain chemicals or drugs.

- Because type A hepatitis usually is spread by the fecal-oral route, a patient with this disease should be on enteric precautions.

- A substantial elevation of the serum transaminase level is characteristic of acute hepatitis.

- For a burn patient, the primary concern is replacement of lost fluid; the secondary concern is infection prevention.

- Excessive vomiting or removal of stomach contents through suction can decrease the potassium level and lead to hypokalemia.

- As a heparin antagonist, protamine sulfate is an antidote for heparin overdose.

- People with obsessive-compulsive disorder realize that their behavior is unreasonable but cannot control it.

- Mannitol (Osmitrol) reduces intracranial pressure by promoting osmotic diuresis.

- If a patient has a positive reaction to a tuberculin skin test, such as the purified protein derivative (PPD) test, the nurse should suspect current or past infection and should ask about a history of TB and the presence of early signs and symptoms of TB, such as low-grade fever, weight loss, night sweats, fatigue, and anorexia.

- Signs and symptoms of acute rheumatic fever include chorea, fever, carditis, migratory polyarthritis, erythema marginatum (rash), and subcutaneous nodules.

- A patient with a history of rheumatic fever should receive prophylactic penicillin therapy before undergoing dental treatment. This therapy helps prevent blood contamination with oral bacteria, which could migrate to the heart valves.

- Fruits are high in fiber and low in protein and should be omitted from a low-residue diet.

- Because postoperative pain varies greatly among individuals, the nurse should use an objective scale to assess and quantify pain.

- The fundamental symptoms of schizophrenia can be grouped into four classifications (known as the four As): associative (thought) disturbance, affective disorder, autism, and ambivalence.

- After MI, most patients can resume sexual activity once they can climb two flights of stairs without fatigue or dyspnea.

- Elderly patients are susceptible to orthostatic hypotension because, with age, the baroreceptors become less sensitive to position changes.

- Kegel exercises require contraction and relaxation of the perineal muscles. They help strengthen pelvic muscles and improve urine control in postpartal patients.

- When witnessing psychiatric patients in a threatening confrontation, the nurse's first action should be to instruct them to move away from each other.

- Symptoms of postpartal depression range from mild postpartal blues to an intense, suicidal, depressive psychosis.

- A preterm neonate may require gavage feedings because of a weak sucking reflex, uncoordinated sucking, or respiratory distress.

- Postmortem care includes cleaning and preparing the deceased patient for family viewing, arranging transportation to the morgue or funeral home, and determining the disposition of belongings.

- For a patient with suspected renal or urethral calculi, the nurse should strain the urine to determine if calculi have been passed.

- The nurse should place a patient with ascites in semi-Fowler's position because it affords maximum lung expansion.

- For a patient who has ingested poison, the nurse should save the vomitus for analysis.

- The nurse should provide honest answers to a patient's questions.

- Acrocyanosis (blueness and coolness of the arms and legs) is normal in neonates because of their immature peripheral circulatory system.

- The earliest signs of respiratory distress are increased respiratory rate followed by increased pulse rate.

- In adults, gastroenteritis usually is self-limiting and produces diarrhea, abdominal discomfort, nausea, and vomiting.

- The patient who has had surgery to correct retinal detachment should avoid sudden movement because it places pressure on the suture line.

- Milk should not be included in a clear liquid diet.

- In patients with acute meningitis, the CSF protein level is elevated.

- When a patient is suspected of having food poisoning, the nurse should notify public health authorities so they can interview patients and food handlers and take samples of the suspected contaminated food.

- A patient receiving a potassium-wasting diuretic should eat potassium-rich foods.

- Consistency in nursing personnel is paramount when caring for a child, an infant, or a confused patient.

- Hypercapnia, marked by an abnormally high carbon dioxide level in the blood, can result from hypoventilation.

- The hypothalamus secretes vasopressin and oxytocin, which are stored in the pituitary gland.

- The three membranes that enclose the brain and spinal cord are the dura mater, pia mater, and arachnoid.

- A nasogastric tube is used to remove fluid and gas from the small intestines in preparation for surgery.

- To prevent ophthalmia neonatorum (a severe eye infection caused by maternal gonorrhea), the nurse may administer one of three medications, as prescribed, in the neonate's eyes: tetracycline, silver nitrate, and erythromycin.

- When a patient is being fitted with crutches, the pressure should be on the hands and not on the axillae because pressure on the axillae can damage the brachial nerve and cause crutch paralysis.

- In metabolic acidosis, a patient may develop Kussmaul's respirations because the rate and depth of respirations increase to "blow off" excess carbonic acids.

- In a female patient, gonorrhea affects the vagina and fallopian tubes.

- Phenylketonuria (PKU) is an inborn error in phenylalanine metabolism, resulting in high serum levels of phenylalanine, cerebral damage, and mental retardation.

- The greatest threats to a patient who has suffered traumatic amputation are blood loss amd hypovolemic shock. Initial interventions should control bleeding and replace fluid and blood as needed.

- Epinephrine hydrochloride is a sympathomimetic drug that acts primarily on alpha, beta$_1$, and beta$_2$ receptors, causing vasoconstriction.

- Epinephrine's adverse effects include dyspnea, tachycardia, palpitations, headaches, and hypertension.

- A psychologist, physical therapist, physician's assistant, or chiropractor is not authorized to write prescriptions for medication.

- The area around a stoma should be cleaned with mild soap and water.

- Vegetables have a high fiber content.

- A cardinal sign of pancreatitis is an elevated serum amylase level.

- During colostomy irrigation, painful cramps usually are caused by too rapid infusion of irrigation solution or infusion of too much solution.

- High colonic irrigation is used to stimulate peristalsis and reduce flatulence.

- The nurse should use a tuberculin syringe to administer a subcutaneous injection of less than 1 ml.

- Bleeding is the most common postoperative problem.

- A patient can control some colostomy odors by not eating such foods as fish, eggs, onions, beans, and cabbages and related vegetables.

- For adults, subcutaneous injections require a 25G, 1" (2.5 cm) needle; for infants, children, or elderly or very thin patients, they require a 25G to 27G, ½" (1.3 cm) needle.

- Before administering medication, the nurse should identify the patient by checking the identification band and asking the patient to state his or her name.

- To clean the skin before an injection, the nurse should use a sterile alcohol swab and wipe from the center of the site outward in a circular motion.

- The nurse always should inject heparin deep into subcutaneous tissue at a 90-degree angle (perpendicular to the skin) to prevent skin irritation.

- If blood is aspirated into the syringe before an I.M. injection, the nurse should withdraw the needle, prepare another syringe, and repeat the procedure.

- The nurse should not cut a patient's hair without written consent from the patient or an appropriate relative.

- If bleeding occurs after an injection, the nurse should apply pressure until the bleeding stops. If bruising occurs, the nurse should monitor the site for an enlarging hematoma.

- When providing hair and scalp care, the nurse should begin combing at the end of the hair and work toward the head.

- Frequency of patient hair care depends on the length and texture of the hair, duration of hospitalization, and patient's condition.

- When paralysis or coma impairs or erases the corneal reflex, frequent eye care aims to keep the exposed cornea moist, preventing ulceration and inflammation.

- Proper hearing aid function requires careful handling during insertion and removal, regular cleaning of the earmold to prevent wax buildup, and prompt replacement of dead batteries.

- The hearing aid marked with a blue dot is for the left ear; the one with the red dot is for the right ear.

- A hearing aid should not be exposed to heat or humidity and should not be immersed in water.

- The nurse should instruct a female patient not to use hair spray while wearing a hearing aid.

- The five branches of pharmacology are pharmacokinetics, pharmacodynamics, pharmacotherapeutics, toxicology, and pharmacognosy.

- Interventions for a patient with AIDS include treating existing infections and cancers, reducing the risk of opportunistic infections, maintaining adequate nutrition and hydration, and providing emotional support to the patient and family.

• A 25-watt bulb should be used for a heat lamp, and the lamp should be placed 18" away from the treatment site.

• Redness from heat lamp use indicates that the patient's skin is being burned. The nurse should remove the lamp and notify the physician.

• The nurse should remove heel protectors every 8 hours to inspect the foot for signs of skin breakdown.

• Signs and symptoms of a chlamydial infection are urinary frequency; thin, white vaginal or urethral discharge; and cervical inflammation.

• The purpose of heat application is to promote vasodilation, which reduces pain caused by inflammation.

• Chlamydial infection is the most prevalent sexually transmitted disease in the United States.

• The pituitary gland is located in the sella turcica of the sphenoid bone in the cranial cavity.

• Myasthenia gravis is a neuromuscular disorder characterized by impulse disturbances at the myoneural junction.

• A sutured surgical incision is an example of healing by first intention (healing directly, without granulation).

• Healing by secondary intention (healing by granulation) is closure of the wound with granulations. The granulation tissue fills the defect and allows re-epithelialization to occur, beginning at the wound edges and continuing to the center, until the entire wound is covered.

• Keloid formation is an abnormality in healing characterized by overgrowth of scar tissue at the wound site.

• Patients with anorexia nervosa or bulimia must be observed during the meal and for a time afterward to ensure that they do not purge after eating.

• Myasthenia gravis usually affects young women, producing these signs and symptoms: extreme muscle weakness and fatigability, difficulty chewing and talking, strabismus, and ptosis.

• Transsexuals believe that they were born the wrong gender and often seek hormonal or surgical treatment to change their gender.

• Tay-Sachs disease results from a congenital enzyme deficiency and is characterized by progressive mental and motor deterioration.

• Hypothermia is a life-threatening disorder in which the body's core temperature drops below 95º F (35º C).

• Treatment of PKU must begin within the first few weeks of life to prevent brain damage.

• Neonatal testing for PKU has become mandatory in most states.

• Although no cure exists for Tay-Sachs disease, serum analysis for hexosaminidase A deficiency allows for accurate identification of genetic carriers of the disease.

• Signs and symptoms of hypopituitarism in adults may include gonadal failure, diabetes insipidus, hypothyroidism, and adrenocortical insufficiency.

• Reiter's syndrome causes a triad of symptoms: arthritis, conjunctivitis, and urethritis.

• Down syndrome (trisomy 21) is the most common chromosomal disorder.

• A carbohydrate-restricted diet for patients who have had a partial gastrectomy provides foods high in protein and fats and restricts foods high in carbohydrates because they are quickly digested and are more readily emptied from the stomach into the duodenum, causing diarrhea.

- The nurse should place a neonate in a 30-degree Trendelenburg position to facilitate mucus drainage.

- The nurse may suction a neonate's nose and mouth as needed with a bulb syringe or suction trap.

- To prevent heat loss, the nurse first should place the neonate under a radiant warmer during suctioning and initial delivery-room care and then should wrap the neonate in a warmed blanket for transport to the nursery.

- The umbilical cord normally has two arteries and one vein.

- When providing care, the nurse should expose only one part of an infant's body at a time.

- *Lightening* refers to the settling of the fetal head into the brim of the pelvis.

- If the neonate is stable, the mother should be allowed to breast-feed within the neonate's first hour of life.

- The nurse should check a neonate's temperature every 1 to 2 hours until it is maintained within normal limits.

- At birth, the neonate normally weighs 5½ to 9 lb (2 to 4.1 kg), measures 18" to 22" (39.6 to 48.4 cm) in length, has a head circumference of 13½" to 14" (29.7 to 30.8 cm), and has a chest circumference that is 1" (2.5 cm) less than the head circumference.

- In a neonate, temperature normally ranges from 98° to 99° F (36.7° to 37.2° C), apical pulse averages 120 to 160 beats/minute, and respirations are 40 to 60 breaths/minute.

- The diamond-shaped anterior fontanel usually closes between ages 12 and 18 months; the triangular posterior fontanel usually closes by age 2 months.

- In a neonate, a straight spine is normal; a tuft of hair over the spine is abnormal.

- Prostaglandin gel may be applied to the vagina or cervix to ripen an unfavorable cervix before labor induction with oxytocin (Pitocin).

- When administering an oral medication to an infant, the nurse should place it in the side of the mouth and encourage swallowing by gently lifting the infant's chin with the thumb and stroking the infant's neck.

- Supernumerary nipples occasionally are seen on neonates and usually appear along a line that runs from each axilla through the normal nipple area to the groin.

- Meconium is a material that collects in the fetus's intestines and forms the neonate's first stools, which are black and tarry.

- The presence of meconium in the amniotic fluid during labor indicates possible fetal distress and the need to evaluate the neonate for meconium aspiration.

- Polydactyly (more than the normal number of fingers or toes) is a congenital anomaly.

- A positive Babinski's reflex (toe fanning when the sole is stroked from heel to toe) is normal in the neonate and may persist for up to 18 months.

- To assess the rooting reflex, the nurse touches a finger to the neonate's cheek or corner of mouth. Normally, the neonate turns the head toward the stimulus, opens the mouth, and searches for the stimulus.

- Harlequin sign is present when a neonate lying on the side appears red on the dependent side and pale on the upper side.

- The nurse should administer procaine penicillin by deep I.M. injection in the upper outer portion of the buttocks in an adult or in the midlateral thigh in a child. The injection site should not be massaged.

- Mongolian spots are slight gray patches across the sacrum, buttocks, and legs. These normal variations are common in non-Caucasian infants and usually disappear by age 2 to 3.

- Vernix caseosa is a cheese-like substance that covers and protects the fetus's skin in utero. It may be rubbed into the neonate's skin or washed away in one or two baths.

- A fugue state is a dissociative state in which a person leaves familiar surroundings, assumes a new identity, and develops amnesia about the previous identity.

- Caput succedaneum is scalp edema that develops during labor and delivery. It resolves spontaneously and presents no danger to the neonate.

- Nevus flammeus, or port-wine stain, is a diffuse pink to dark bluish red lesion on a neonate's face or neck.

- Strawberry hemangiomas are raised red birthmarks that may continue to spread up to age 1. Complete shrinkage and absorption of hemangiomas may take 7 to 10 years.

- Cavernous hemangiomas resemble strawberry hemangiomas but do not disappear with age.

- The Guthrie test (a screening test for PKU) is most reliable if it is done between the 2nd and 6th days after birth and after the neonate has ingested protein.

- To assess coordination of sucking and swallowing, the nurse should observe a neonate's first breast-feeding or bottle-feeding with sterile water.

- To establish a milk supply pattern, a mother should breast-feed her infant at least every 4 hours; during the 1st month, she should breast-feed 8 to 12 times a day (demand feeding).

- The nurse should wear gloves when handling a neonate until after the first bath is given.

- For an infant with a suspected infection, the nurse should maintain isolation and take other appropriate precautions.

- If a breast-fed infant is content and has good skin turgor, an adequate number of wet diapers, and normal weight gain, the mother's milk supply is considered adequate.

- For a female patient of child-bearing age who is undergoing chemotherapy, the nurse should encourage the use of a contraceptive during sexual intercourse because of the risk of fetal damage if she becomes pregnant.

- Pernicious anemia is vitamin B_{12} deficiency caused by a lack of intrinsic factor, which is produced by the gastric mucosal parietal cells.

- To perform pursed-lip breathing, the patient inhales through the nose and exhales slowly and evenly against pursed lips while contracting the abdominal muscles.

- The ascending colostomy drains fluid feces; the descending colostomy drains solid fecal matter.

- A patient undergoing chemotherapy should consume a high-calorie, high-protein diet.

- Adverse effects of chemotherapy include bone marrow depression, which causes anemia, leukopenia, and thrombocytopenia; GI epithelial cell irritation, which causes GI ulceration, bleeding, and vomiting; and destruction of hair follicles and skin, which causes alopecia and dermatitis.

- An infant with celiac disease has fatty, foul-smelling stools.

- The hemoglobin electrophoresis test differentiates between sickle cell trait and sickle cell anemia.

- A folded towel can provide scrotal support for a patient with scrotal edema caused by vasectomy, epididymitis, or orchitis.

- In the supine position, a pregnant patient's enlarged uterus impairs venous return from the lower half of the body to the heart, resulting in supine hypotensive syndrome.

- Treatment of ankle edema in a pregnant patient consists of frequent rest periods, foot elevation, and avoidance of constricting clothing, such as garters and pantyhose.

- Erythromycin, clindamycin, and tetracycline produce their antibiotic effects by inhibiting protein synthesis in susceptible organisms.

- *Eruption* refers to the normal presentation of a tooth as it penetrates the gum.

- Recommended weight gain during pregnancy is 25 to 35 lb (11.3 to 15.8 kg).

- The nurse administers oxygen as prescribed to a patient with CHF to help overcome hypoxia and dyspnea.

- Signs and symptoms of small-bowel obstruction include decreased or absent bowel sounds, abdominal distention, decreased flatus, and projectile vomiting.

- The nurse should use both hands when ventilating a patient with an Ambu bag. (One hand can deliver only 400 cc of air; two hands can deliver 1,000 cc of air.)

- Dosages of methylxanthine agents, such as theophylline (Theo-Dur) and aminophylline (Aminophyllin), should be individualized based on serum drug level, patient response, and adverse reactions.

- When determining which information to give a hospitalized child about a procedure, the nurse should consider the child's developmental—not chronologic—age.

- The patient should apply a transdermal scopolamine patch (Transderm-Scop) at least 4 hours before its antiemetic action is needed.

• Early indications of gangrene are edema, pain, redness, tissue darkening, and coldness in the affected body part.

• Ipecac syrup is the emetic of choice because of its effectiveness in evacuating the stomach and relatively low incidence of adverse reactions.

• When giving an injection to a patient with a bleeding disorder, the nurse should use a small-gauge needle and apply pressure to the site for 5 minutes after the injection.

• Platelets are the smallest and most fragile formed element of the blood and are essential for coagulation.

• To insert a nasogastric tube, the nurse should first instruct the patient to tilt the head back slightly and then insert the tube. When the tube is felt curving at the pharynx, the nurse should tell the patient to tilt the head forward to close the trachea and open the esophagus.

• The nurse should inform a patient taking oral iron (ferrous sulfate) that it may color the stools dark green to black.

• Polycythemia vera causes pruritus, painful fingers and toes, hyperuricemia, plethora (reddish purple skin and mucosa), weakness, and easy fatigability.

• Rheumatic fever usually is preceded by a group A beta-hemolytic streptococcal infection, such as scarlet fever, otitis media, streptococcal throat infection, impetigo, or tonsillitis.

• A thyroid storm or crisis, an extreme form of hyperthyroidism, is characterized by hyperpyrexia with a temperature of up to 106° F (41.1° C), diarrhea, dehydration, tachycardia up to 200 beats/minute, arrhythmias, extreme irritability, and delirium. It may lead to coma, shock, and death.

• Tardive dyskinesia, an adverse reaction to long-term psychotropic drug use, produces involuntary repetitive movements of the tongue, lips, extremities, and trunk.

- Tocolytic agents used to treat preterm labor include terbutaline sulfate (Brethine), ritodrine hydrochloride (Yutopar), and magnesium sulfate.

- A pregnant woman with hyperemesis gravidarum may require hospitalization to treat dehydration and starvation.

- *Asthma* refers to bronchoconstriction in response to allergens, such as food, pollen, or drugs; irritants, such as smoke or paint fumes; infections; weather changes; exercise; or gastroesophageal reflex. In the United States, about 5% of children have chronic asthma.

- Diaphragmatic hernia is one of the most urgent neonatal surgical emergencies. By compressing and displacing the lungs and heart, this disorder can cause respiratory distress to occur shortly after birth.

- Blood cultures help identify the cause of endocarditis; an increased WBC count suggests bacterial infection.

- Common complications of early pregnancy (up to 20 weeks' gestation) include fetal loss or serious threats to maternal health.

- For a patient with an acute aortic dissection, the nursing priority is to maintain the mean arterial pressure between 60 and 65. A vasodilator, such as nitroprusside sodium (Nipride), may be needed to achieve this.

- For a patient with congestive heart failure, one of the most important nursing diagnoses is *Pain related to imbalance between oxygen supply and demand.*

- For a patient receiving peritoneal dialysis, the nurse must monitor body weight and BUN, creatinine, and electrolyte levels.

- ACE inhibitors, such as captopril (Capoten) and enalapril (Vasotec), decrease blood pressure by interfering with the renin-angiotensin-aldosterone system.

- A patient with stable ventricular tachycardia has a blood pressure and is conscious. Therefore, the patient's cardiac output is being maintained, and the nurse must monitor vital signs continuously.

- ACE inhibitors inhibit the enzyme that converts angiotensin I into angiotensin II, which is a potent vasoconstrictor. Through this action, they reduce peripheral arterial resistance and blood pressure.

- When caring for a patient receiving a diuretic, the nurse should monitor serum electrolyte levels, check vital signs, and observe for orthostatic hypotension.

- According to families whose loved ones are in critical care units, their four most important needs are to have questions answered honestly, to be assured that the best possible care is being provided, to know the prognosis, and to feel there is hope.

- Breast self-examination (BSE) is one of the most important health habits to teach a female patient. It should be done on the 5th to 7th day after the 1st day of the menstrual period because that is when hormonal effects, which can cause breast lumps and tenderness, are reduced.

- Postmenopausal women should choose a regular time each month to perform BSE.

- In a postmenopausal woman receiving cyclical estrogen, the best time for BSE is the last day that she is not taking the estrogen.

- When preparing a patient for chest tube removal, the nurse should explain that it may cause pain or a burning or pulling sensation.

- Essential hypertensive renal disease usually is characterized by progressive renal impairment.

Notes

_____

_____

_____

_____

_____

_____

_____

_____

_____

_____

_____

_____

_____

_____

_____

_____

_____

_____

_____

_____

_____

Notes